Helminth control in school-age children

A guide for managers
of control programmes

Second edition

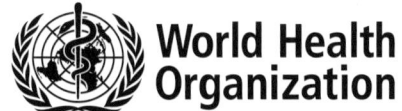

World Health Organization

WHO Library Cataloguing-in-Publication Data:

Helminth control in school age children: a guide for managers of control programmes - 2nd ed.

1. Helminthiasis - prevention and control 2. Helminthiasis - drug therapy. 3.Schistosomiasis - prevention and control 4.Schistosomiasis -drug therapy. 5.Helminths - growth and development. 6.Anthelmintics - therapeutic use. 7.Child. 8.National health programs - organization and administration 9.Guidelines. I.World Health Organization.

ISBN 978 92 4 154826 7   (NLM classification: WC 800)

First edition, 2002
Seconedition, 2011

Design, Layout: Patrick Tissot, WHO/HTM/NTD

Printed in France

Contents > Highlights

Helminth control in school-age children • Second edition

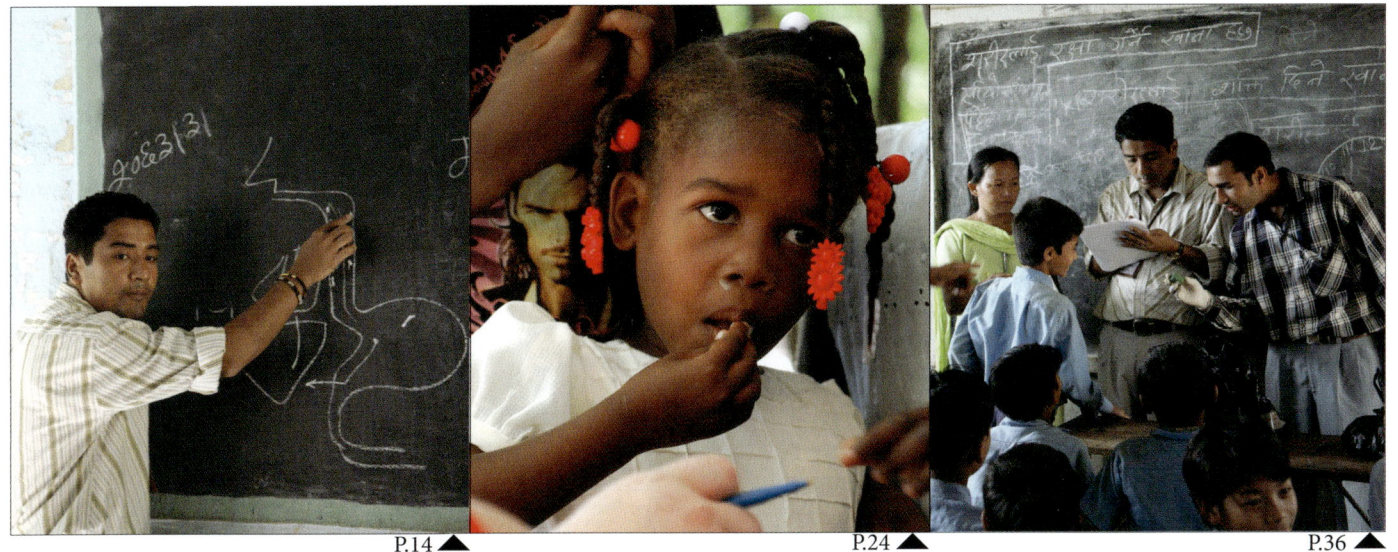

P.14 ▲   P.24 ▲   P.36 ▲

Contents

Inside Back cover: Tablet pole for dosing praziquantel

Preface

IN 2001, THE WORLD HEALTH ASSEMBLY,
with Resolution 54.19, set the global target of treatment of 75% of school-age children (usually defined as children between 5 and 14 years) at risk for schistosomiasis and soil-transmitted helminth (STH) infections by 2010. WHO estimates that more than 200 million school-age children were treated worldwide in 2009.

The purpose of this book is to offer guidance to planners and programme managers in the health and education sectors with responsibility for these control programmes and to provide encouragement to those who will be instrumental in achieving this global target.

The school-based control of schistosomiasis and STH infections is of proven cost effectiveness. This book describes an approach in which epidemiological data are used to select the control strategy to be applied to the school-age population and shows how periodic data collection from sentinel sites can be used to monitor the progress of control activities.

The first edition of this book was published in 2002. This second edition incorporates more recent experience and lessons learnt from school-based control programmes in several countries not previously reported. It also includes references to web sites where useful information is available.

The book is intended to help managers plan, implement and monitor programmes for deworming school-age children using methods based on the best current evidence and experience. It covers the following topics:

- A summary of the relevant health risks caused by schistosomiasis and STH infections, modes of transmission of the infections and public health measures that can be applied to control the risks.

- Guiding principles for school health programme design and budgeting, including details of procurement of drugs and other materials and of the organization of training activities.

- Guiding principles for the implementation of school health programmes, including logistics management in the school system, the administration of deworming drugs to the children and the management of adverse events.

- Suggestion for the integration of schistosomiasis and STH control activities with onchocerciasis and filariasis control/elimination programmes in the context of the national control of neglected tropical diseases.

- The most useful indicators for monitoring and evaluating the progress of the programme, including guidelines for the collection of epidemiological data and for reducing the frequency of drug administration.

WHO is currently supporting endemic countries in preparing integrated plans for control of neglected tropical diseases in which these aspects are considered. Managers of control programmes should contact WHO's Department of Control of Neglected Tropical Diseases (see list of useful addresses in *Annex 1*) for support and for information about integrated control.

Control and the sustainable interruption of transmission will depend on the successful implementation of deworming programmes and on intersectoral collaboration to improve basic hygiene and living conditions.

Nine examples from existing school health programmes are presented to illustrate specific aspects of the deworming intervention. This book is a source of guidance; regional and national factors will influence the actual control strategies to be implemented; the illustrative examples are a means of sharing practical and specific experience.

Acknowledgements

Helminth control in school-age children • Second edition

THE WORLD HEALTH ORGANIZATION WOULD LIKE to express special thanks to all those who contributed to the production of this manual.

The writing committee comprised the following individuals:

Dr Antonio Montresor, Control of Neglected Tropical Diseases, WHO, Geneva, Switzerland

Dr Marco Albonico, Ivo de Carneri Foundation, Milan, Italy

Dr Meklit Berhan, Children Without Worms, Atlanta, GA, USA

Dr Lester Chitsulo, Control of Neglected Tropical Diseases, WHO, Geneva, Switzerland

Professor David Crompton, University of Glasgow, Glasgow, Scotland

Dr Abdoulaye Diarra, WHO Inter-country Support Team for Central Africa, Libreville, Gabon

Dr Dirk Engels, Control of Neglected Tropical Diseases, WHO, Geneva, Switzerland

Dr Albis Gabrielli, Control of Neglected Tropical Diseases, WHO, Geneva, Switzerland.

Professor Theresa W. Gyorkos, McGill University, Montreal, Canada

Dr Pamela Mbabazi, Control of Neglected Tropical Diseases, WHO, Geneva, Switzerland

Dr Eric Ottesen, Emory University, Atlanta, USA

Dr Lorenzo Savioli, Control of Neglected Tropical Diseases, WHO, Geneva, Switzerland

Dr Aya Yajima, Control of Neglected Tropical Diseases, WHO, Geneva, Switzerland

Thanks are due to the following people for their contributions, suggestions and support:

Dr Simon Brooker, KEMRI-Wellcome Trust Research Programme, Kenya

Professor Nilanthi de Silva, University of Kelaniya, Kelaniya, Sri Lanka

Dr Jonathan D. King, The Carter Center, Atlanta, GA, USA

Ms Kim Koporc, Children Without Worms, Atlanta, GA, USA

Dr Patrick Lammie, Centers for Disease Control and Prevention, Atlanta, GA, USA

Ms Seung Lee, Save the Children US, Washington, DC, USA

Dr Frank O. Richards Jr. , The Carter Center, Atlanta, GA, USA

Dr Francesco Rio, Control of Neglected Tropical Diseases, WHO, Geneva, Switzerland

Mrs Natalie Roschnik, Save the Children US, Washington, DC, USA

Dr Muth Sinuon, National Malaria Center, Ministry of Health of Cambodia, Phnom Penh, Cambodia

Grateful acknowledgement is also due to the United States Agency for International Development (USAID) and the Global Network for Neglected Tropical Diseases (GNNTD) for financial assistance with the publication of this document.

Glossary

Helminth control in school-age children • Second edition

THE DEFINITIONS PROVIDED HERE RELATE TO THE use of terms in this book and may not necessarily be valid in other contexts.

adverse event (AE)
Any untoward medical occurrence that may present during treatment with a medicine but that does not necessarily have a causal relationship with this treatment. (See also adverse drug reaction.)

adverse drug reaction (ADR)
A response to a drug which is noxious and unintended and which occurs at drug doses indicated for use in humans. (See also serious adverse event.)

anaemia
Clinical condition reflecting an inadequate number of red blood cells or an insufficient amount of haemoglobin (Hb) in the blood. Children aged 5–11 years are considered to be anaemic when the Hb concentration is below 115 g/litre and severely anaemic when it is below 80 g/litre. Children aged 12–14 years are considered to be anaemic when the Hb concentration is below 120 g/litre and severely anaemic when it is below 80 g/litre.

ascites
See hepatosplenomegaly.

cercaria
See life cycle of schistosomes.

coverage
The proportion of the target population reached by an intervention (e.g. percentage of school-age children treated on a treatment day).

cure rate (CR)
Percentage of infected individuals in a community who, after treatment, are no longer infected (usually determined on the basis of a negative stool specimen).

deworming round
Distribution of an anthelminthic medicine to a large group of individuals during one defined time period. The deworming activities cannot usually all be conducted simultaneously, so it make take 1–2 weeks or more for a "round" to be completed in a specific target population.

disability-adjusted life years (DALYs)
The number of years of healthy life lost attributable to a disease (or group of diseases). DALYs are used as a measure of disease burden and provide a comparative indication of the public health importance of the disease(s).

disease burden
The cumulative mortality, morbidity and disability attributable to a disease.

dysentery
Frequent discharge of watery stools containing blood and mucus.

ecological zone
See homogeneous ecological zone.

egg reduction rate (ERR)
The difference in mean **eggs per gram (epg)** counts following an intervention (e.g. deworming) in a population. The post-intervention mean epg count is compared with a baseline, or pre-intervention, mean epg count. It is expressed as a percentage (1 - mean post-deworming epg/mean pre-deworming epg).

eggs per gram (epg)
The number of parasite eggs per gram of faeces, which provides an indirect measure of the intensity of helminth infection. (*See also* intensity of infection).

endemic area
Area in which a disease is intensively transmitted.

fibrosis
The formation of fibrous tissue as a reparative or reactive process. Fibrosis of the liver leading to portal hypertension is frequent in *Schistosoma mansoni* and *S. japonicum* infections. (*See also* hepatosplenomegaly).

fluency

The capacity of a person to communicate orally. The fluency test is one of many tests used to measure the level of cognition. It is conducted, for example, by asking the subject to name as many animals as possible in a defined period of time. The task involves both the central executive component of working memory and the long-term semantic memory.

granuloma

Focal lesion resulting from an inflammatory reaction caused, in the case of schistosomiasis, by the eggs of schistosomes. (*See also* hepatosplenomegaly).

haematuria

Presence of red blood cells in the urine. **Visible haematuria** refers to blood present in sufficient quantity to be detectable by visual inspection of the urine sample (the colour of the urine is red-brown). **Microhaematuria** refers to blood that is present in insufficient quantity to be visible to the naked eye but that is detectable using a reagent strip.

haemoglobin (Hb)

The protein contained in red blood cells that transports oxygen to the tissues and organs of the body.

helminthiasis

A general term for any form of disease attributable to a helminth infection. *See also* morbidity.

helminths

A group of parasites commonly referred to as worms. The group includes the trematodes (flukes), cestodes (tapeworms) and nematodes (roundworms). The helminth species covered by this manual are **schistosomes** (trematodes) and **soil-transmitted helminths** (nematodes).

hepatosplenomegaly

Enlargement of the liver and the spleen due, in the case of intestinal schistosomiasis, to the reaction to parasite eggs (**granuloma**). This condition interferes with blood circulation in the two organs and causes portal hypertension (high blood pressure in the venous system entering the liver) and ascites (accumulation of serous fluid in the abdominal cavity). Hepatosplenomegaly and ascites can result in a considerable enlargement of the abdomen ("big belly").

homogeneous ecological zone

Geographical area that is homogeneous in terms of humidity, rainfall, vegetation, population density and sanitation level.

indirect costs of intervention

In the case of deworming of school-age children, the value of the time spent by teachers, as well as by health personnel at central, provincial and district levels, providing deworming as part of their routine work. Such economic costs do not imply any monetary transaction.

intensity of infection

The number of helminths infecting an individual. In the case of soil-transmitted helminths, it can be measured *directly*, by counting expelled worms after anthelminthic treatment, or *indirectly*, by counting helminth eggs excreted in faeces (expressed as eggs per gram, **epg**). Indirect methods are less intrusive, more convenient and more commonly used. In urine, the number of schistosome eggs per 10 ml are counted.

intestinal obstruction

Blockage of the lumen of the intestine. This is a severe complication of ascariasis that occurs in young children and requires surgical intervention.

KAP survey

An assessment of the knowledge, attitudes and practices of a community or group of individuals at one point in time, usually with respect to a health or health-related topic.

larvae

See life cycle of soil-transmitted helminths and schistosomes.

life cycle of schistosomes

Adult schistosomes live in the blood system and produce eggs which are expelled in the faeces or urine of the host. **Miracidia** hatch from eggs excreted in fresh water. The miracidia are mobile in water and infect snails (intermediate host). Infected snails release great quantities of free-swimming larvae (**cercariae**), which can penetrate the skin of humans (definitive host). The cercariae then migrate in the body and transform progressively into adult schistosomes.

life cycle of soil-transmitted helminths

Adult soil-transmitted helminths live in the intestine of the host and produce eggs which are expelled with the host's faeces and contaminate the environment. After a period of maturation the parasite eggs hatch, as infective larvae, in the soil (hookworms) or, after ingestion, in the intestinal tract (*Ascaris lumbricoides* and *Trichuris trichiura*). After penetration of the skin or the digestive mucosa, the larvae of hookworms and *A. lumbricoides* then migrate in the human body, passing from the trachea to the oesophagus and re-entering the intestine where they develop into adult parasites. The larvae of *T. trichiura* develop from the ingested egg into the adult form of the parasite in the intestine, without migrating.

lottery method
Method of sampling in which all the units are equally likely to be selected. For example, the name of each district is written on individual pieces of paper; all papers are placed in a container; and, without looking, one is drawn out at random. (*See also* random sampling.)

malabsorption
Reduced capacity to absorb nutrients through the gastrointestinal tract.

microhaematuria
See haematuria.

micronutrients
Essential nutrients found in food that are required by the human body only in small amounts (e.g. iron, iodine, vitamins).

miracidium
Larval form of the schistosome. *See* life cycle of schistosomes.

morbidity
Clinical consequences of infections and diseases that adversely affect an individual's health. In the case of helminth infection, morbidity can be overt (e.g. **haematuria**, diarrhoea or **ascites**) or subtle (e.g. **malabsorption**, **anaemia**, stunted growth).

neglected tropical diseases (NTDs)
Group of diseases that are considered not to have received sufficient attention from the donor community and public health planners. WHO is currently focusing on the following NTDs: dracunculiasis, lymphatic filariasis, onchocerciasis, schistosomiasis, soil-transmitted helminthiases, Buruli ulcer, Chagas disease, dengue, endemic treponematoses, human African trypanosomiasis, leishmaniasis, leprosy and trachoma. The first five of the diseases in this list are caused by infection with **helminths**.

obstructive uropathy
Structural or functional obstacle to the normal flow of urine. In the case of schistosomiasis, this is due to the presence of **granulomas** in the mucosa of the urogenital system.

outreach activities
Activities designed to provide populations not normally covered by a prevention or control programme (such as non-enrolled school-age children in areas where control programmes are targeted to school-age children) with the same health benefits as those who are covered by the programme.

polymorphism
The ability of a substance to exist in different spatial arrangements of the same chemical elements. Mebendazole exists in three polymorphs (A, B and C).

portal hypertension
See hepatosplenomegaly.

preschool-age children
Children between 1 and 4 years of age.

prevalence of any soil-transmitted helminth infection
The percentage of individuals in a population infected with at least one species of soil-transmitted helminth.

prevalence of infection
Percentage of individuals in a population who are infected. (*See also* prevalence of any soil-transmitted helminth infection.)

preventive chemotherapy
The use of anthelminthic drugs, either alone or in combination, as a public health tool against helminth infections. Preventive chemotherapy can be applied with different modalities:

- *Mass drug administration (MDA)*. The entire population of an area (e.g. state, region, province, district, subdistrict, village) is given anthelminthic drugs at regular intervals, irrespective of the individual infection status.
- *Targeted chemotherapy*. Specific risk groups in the population, defined by age, sex or other social characteristic such as occupation (e.g. school-age children, fishermen) are given anthelminthic drugs at regular intervals, irrespective of the individual infection status.
- *Selective chemotherapy*. After a regular screening exercise in a population group living in an endemic area, all individuals found (or suspected) to be infected are given anthelminthic drugs.

In the control of schistosomiasis or soil-transmitted helminthiases, preventive chemotherapy (i.e. deworming) is mainly targeted at school-age children.

random sampling
The selection of a subset of a population, where the process of selection is by chance. (*See also* lottery method.)

rectal prolapse
Medical condition in which the wall of the rectum protrudes through the anus and become visible outside the body. This is a complication of heavy *T. trichiura* infection.

sanitation
Means of promoting health through prevention of contact with the hazards of human wastes including facilities for the safe disposal of human excreta.

schistosomes
The schistosome species that infect humans are: *Schistosoma haematobium, S. mansoni, S. japonicum, S. mekongi, S. intercalatum* and *S. guineensis*.

schistosomiasis
Parasitic disease caused by schistosomes.

school-age children
Usually defined as children between 5 and 14 years of age who may or may not be enrolled in school. The exact ages of school enrolment can vary slightly between different countries. Because peak prevalence and intensity of schistosome and soil-transmitted helminth infection occur primarily in school-age children, and because this risk population is easily accessed through schools, deworming activities are implemented through the school system. If the school age is different (for example, from 6 to 15 years) in a particular country, this population would be the target of the school deworming activities (see Example 9 in Chapter 5).

serious adverse event (SAE)
An event that is fatal, life-threatening, disabling or results in hospitalization after drug intake.

soil-transmitted helminthiases
Parasitic diseases attributable to soil-transmitted helminths.

soil-transmitted helminths
Four species of nematodes are collectively referred to as "soil-transmitted helminths": the roundworm, *Ascaris lumbricoides*; the whipworm, *Trichuris trichiura*; and the hookworms *Necator americanus* and *Ancylostoma duodenale*.

visible haematuria
See haematuria.

uropathy
A pathological condition involving the urinary tract.

Schistosomiasis and STH infections are diseases of poverty. These infections give rise to much suffering and death; in addition, they contribute to the perpetuation of poverty by impairing the physical and intellectual growth of children, and by diminishing the work capacity and productivity of adults.

Photograph by Brad Wong

BACKGROUND

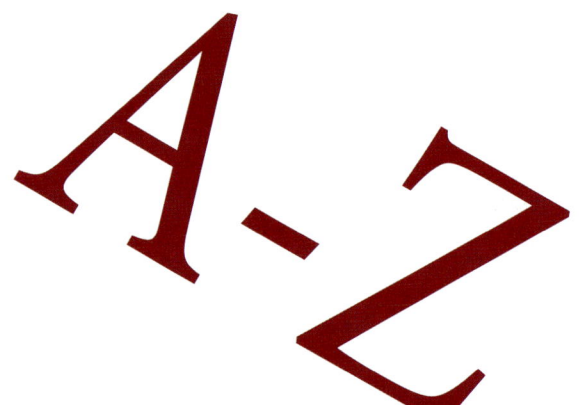

1.1 Schistosomiasis and soil-transmitted helminth infections in the context of neglected tropical diseases

Neglected tropical diseases (NTDs) thrive where there is poverty and disadvantage. Those most affected are the poorest populations, often living in remote, rural areas, in urban slums or in conflict zones: several NTDs are usually transmitted in the same area.[1] Recent estimates suggest that the global burden of NTDs is at least as high as that of malaria or tuberculosis (Hotez et al., 2009).

Several of the NTDs, including schistosomiasis and STH infections, lymphatic filariasis and onchocerciasis, can be controlled easily through the periodic administration of preventive chemotherapy (WHO, 2006).

Use of the school infrastructure to administer deworming drugs is one of the simplest approaches to treating large numbers of school-age children, and school-based programmes have become one of the cornerstones of NTD control.

These guidelines focus on control strategies for the helminth species presented in *Table 1.1*. Strategies for controlling onchocerciasis and lymphatic filariasis are excluded from these guidelines because the control approach is not school-based and specific intervention strategies are adequately covered elsewhere.[2]

1.2 Burden due to schistosomiasis and soil-transmitted helminth infections

It is estimated that more than 2000 million people are affected by schistosomiasis and STH infections worldwide, of whom more than 300 million suffer from associated severe morbidity (de Silva et al., 2003). Global estimates of prevalence, morbidity and mortality are summarized in *Table 1.2*; *Figures 1.1* and *1.2* show the geographical distribution of STH infections and schistosomiasis.

---

[1] For a full description of the diseases covered by WHO's Department of Control of Neglected Tropical Diseases refer to http://www.who.int/neglected_diseases/en/

[2] Most of the training documents for implementation of strategies for the elimination of lymphatic filariasis are available at http://www.who.int/lymphatic_filariasis/resources/en/. Most of the training documents for implementation of strategies for onchocerciasis control are available at http://www.who.int/apoc/publications/en/

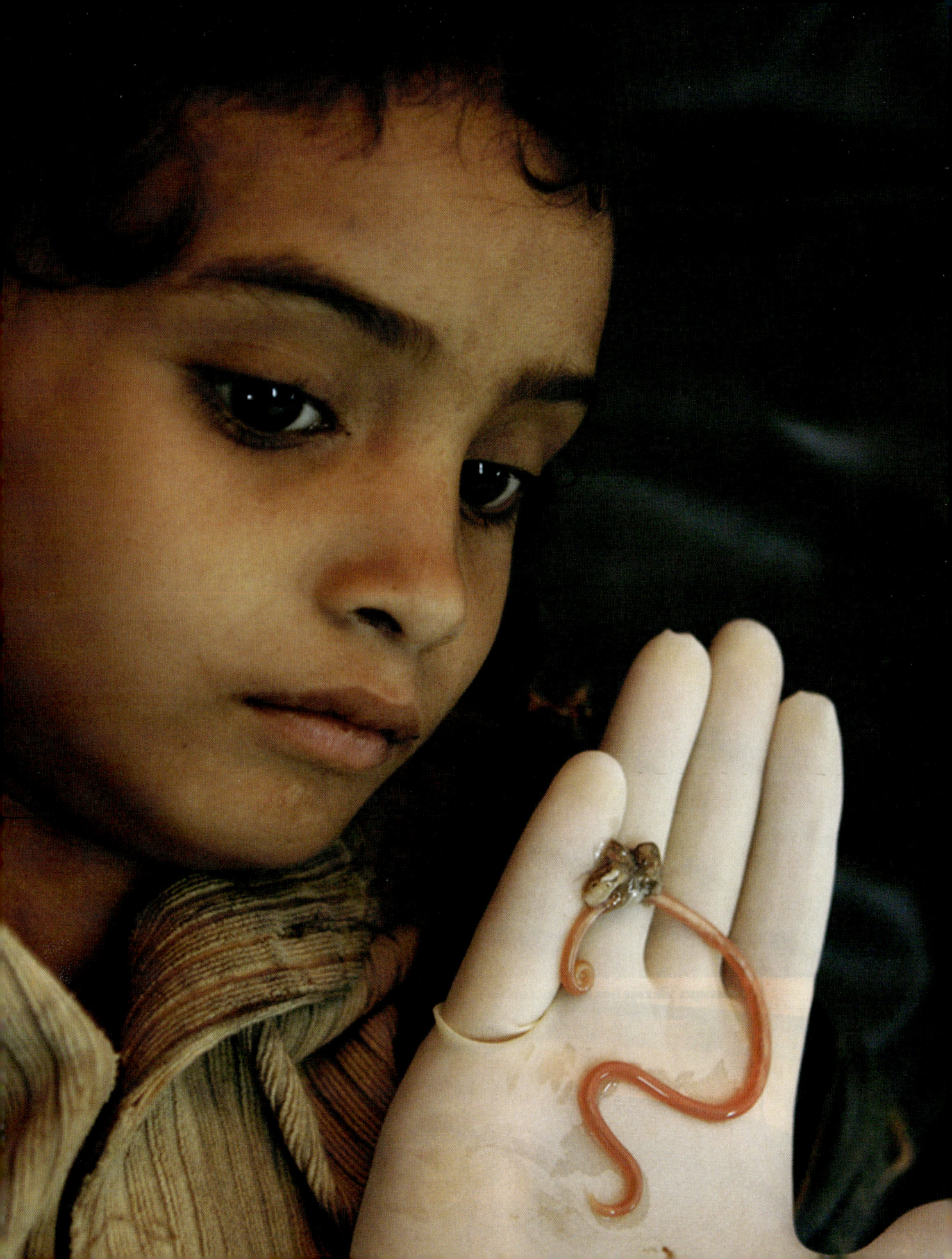

Table 1.1 Helminth species of concern in these guidelines

	Parasite species	**Common name**
Schistosomes	*Schistosoma japonicum* *Schistosoma mansoni* *Schistosoma mekongi*	Intestinal blood flukes
	Schistosoma haematobium	Urinary blood fluke
Soil-transmitted helminths	*Ascaris lumbricoides*	Roundworm
	Ancylostoma duodenale *Necator americanus*	Hookworms*
	Trichuris trichiura	Whipworm

* *A. duodenale* and *N. americanus* are frequently reported together because their eggs are indistinguishable by microscopy.

Table 1.2 Estimates of global morbidity expressed in disability-adjusted life years (DALYs) and mortality due to schistosomiasis and STH infections*

Parasite infections and diseases caused by:	**No. infected (millions)**	**DALYs lost (millions)**	**Mortality (thousands)**
Soil-transmitted helminths			
A. lumbricoides	800	1.2–10.5	3–60
hookworms (*A. duodenale, N. americanus*)	600	1.8–22.1	3–65
T. trichiura	600	1.6–6.4	3–10
Schistosomes	200	1.7–4.5	15–280

* Adapted from Hotez et al, 2009.

Soil-transmitted helminth infections are widely distributed in tropical and sub-tropical areas. In contrast, schistosome infections occur much more focally, depending on local environmental conditions and on the presence of water and an intermediate host (susceptible species of snail).

1.3 Transmission and morbidity

1.3.1 Transmission

Schistosomes and STH are transmitted by eggs excreted in human faeces or urine which contaminate the soil and water sources in areas that lack adequate sanitation. Humans are infected through:

- ingestion of infective eggs (*Ascaris lumbricoides* and *Trichuris trichiura*) or larvae (*Ancylostoma duodenale*) contaminating food, hands or utensils;
- penetration of the skin by infective larvae contaminating the soil (hookworms) or fresh water (schistosomes).

Since these parasites do not multiply in the human host, reinfection occurs only as a result of contact with infective stages in the environment (see *Figures 1.3* and *1.4*).

Figure 1.1 Global distribution of soil-transmitted helminth (STH) infections. Proportion of children requiring preventive chemotherapy for STH in each country.

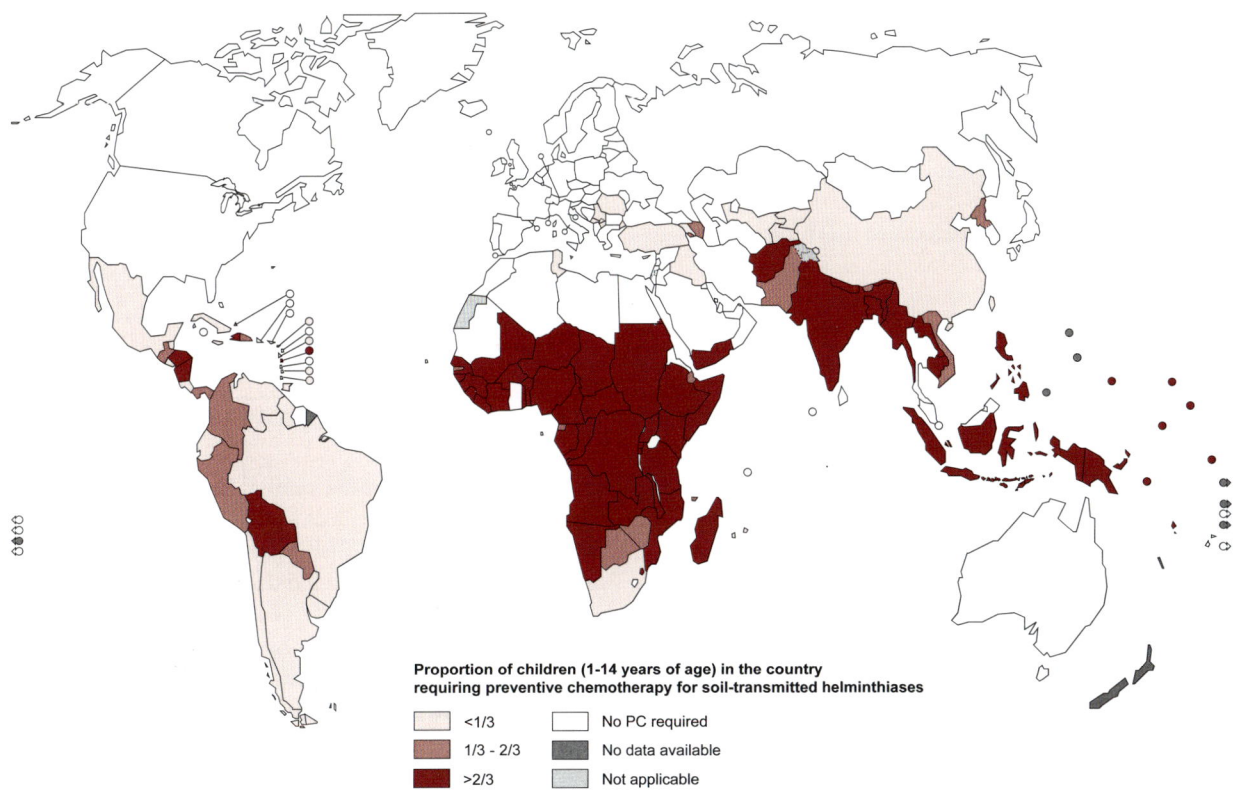

Proportion of children (1-14 years of age) in the country requiring preventive chemotherapy for soil-transmitted helminthiases

- <1/3
- 1/3 - 2/3
- >2/3
- No PC required
- No data available
- Not applicable

Figure 1.2 Global distribution of schistosomiasis.

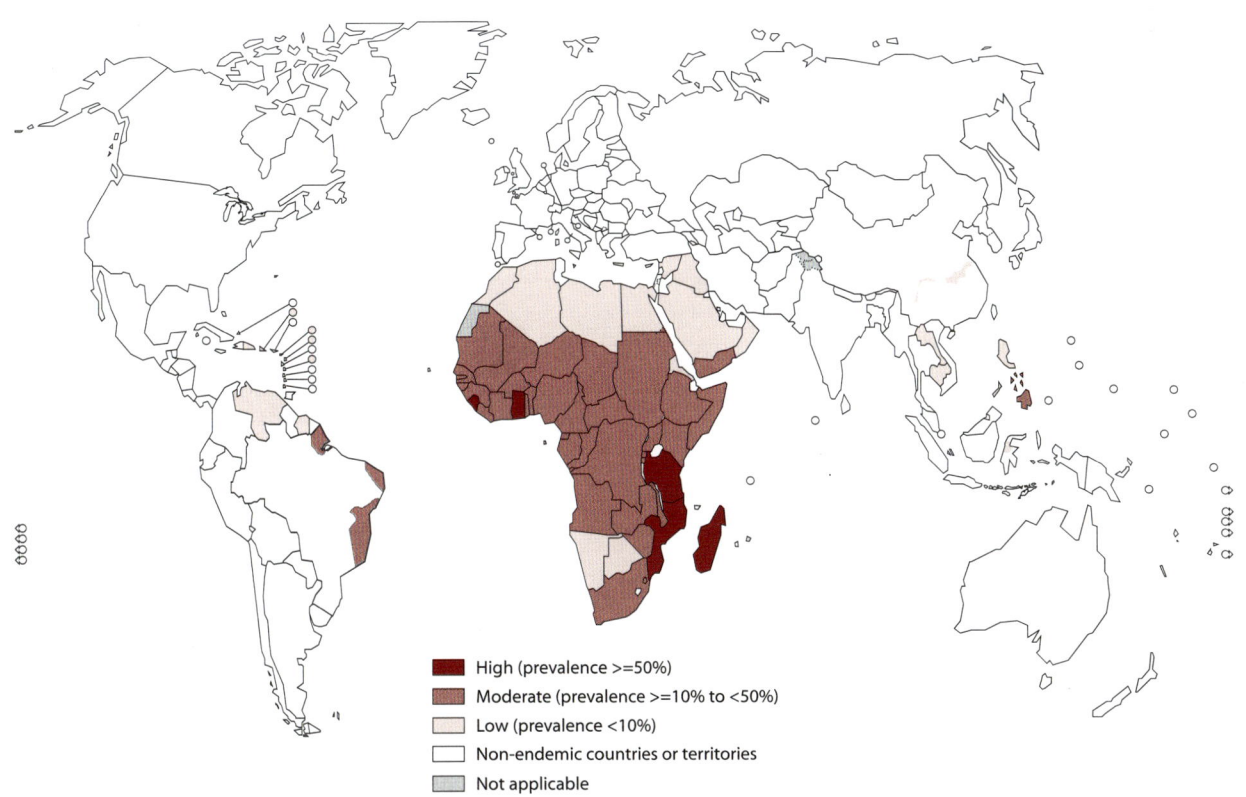

- High (prevalence >=50%)
- Moderate (prevalence >=10% to <50%)
- Low (prevalence <10%)
- Non-endemic countries or territories
- Not applicable

1.3.2 Morbidity

Morbidity is directly related to worm burden: the greater the number of worms in the infected person, the greater will be the severity of disease. In the case of hookworms, for example, the amount of blood lost in the faeces (as an indicator of morbidity) increases as the number of worms (measured in terms of eggs per gram of faeces) increases.

Schistosomiasis and STH infections cause morbidity, and sometimes death, by:

- adversely affecting nutritional status;
- impairing cognitive processes;
- causing complications that require surgical intervention;
- inducing reactions in tissues (notably granuloma).

Schistosomiasis and STH infections are diseases of poverty. These infections give rise to much suffering and death; in addition, they contribute to the perpetuation of poverty by impairing the physical and intellectual growth of children, and by diminishing the work capacity and productivity of adults.

Common examples of morbidity caused by schistosomiasis and STH infections in humans are shown in *Table 1.3*. Concomitant infections with other parasite species are frequent (Keiser et al., 2002; Brito et al., 2006) and may have an additive effect on nutritional status and organ pathology (Pullan & Brooker, 2008).

Infections of heavy intensity are the major cause of morbidity.

1.4 Essential epidemiological data for control

Epidemiological data are essential to understanding the relevance of schistosomiasis and STH infections in a community and to establishing control measures. Two kinds of data are normally collected during surveys:

A. *Prevalence of infection* is a measure of the number of infected people in a community. In the case of STH, the prevalence of infection *with any of the STH parasites* indicates the percentage of infected children.

Figure 1.3 Schematic life-cycle of soil-transmitted helminths

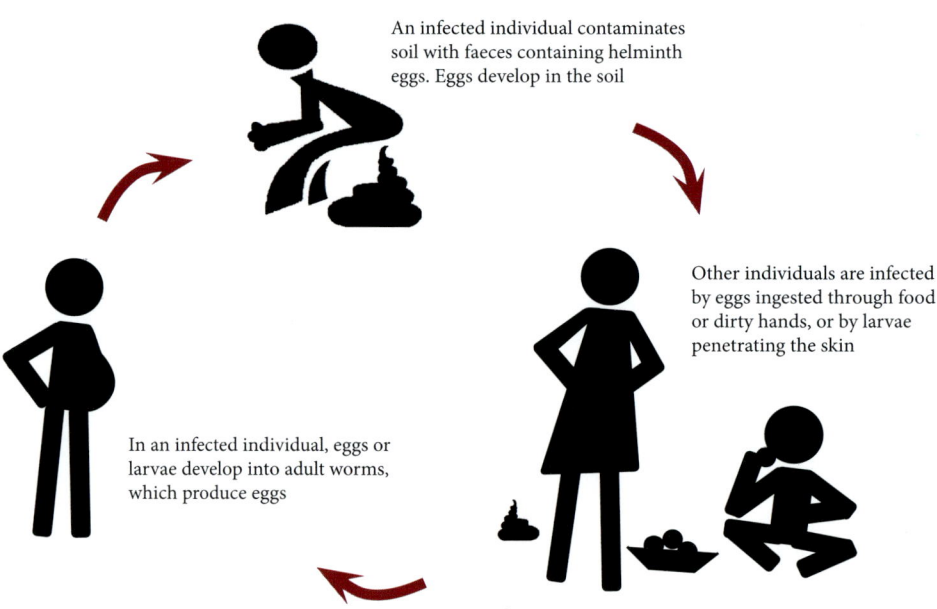

An infected individual contaminates soil with faeces containing helminth eggs. Eggs develop in the soil

Other individuals are infected by eggs ingested through food or dirty hands, or by larvae penetrating the skin

In an infected individual, eggs or larvae develop into adult worms, which produce eggs

Figure 1.4 Schematic life-cycle of schistosomes

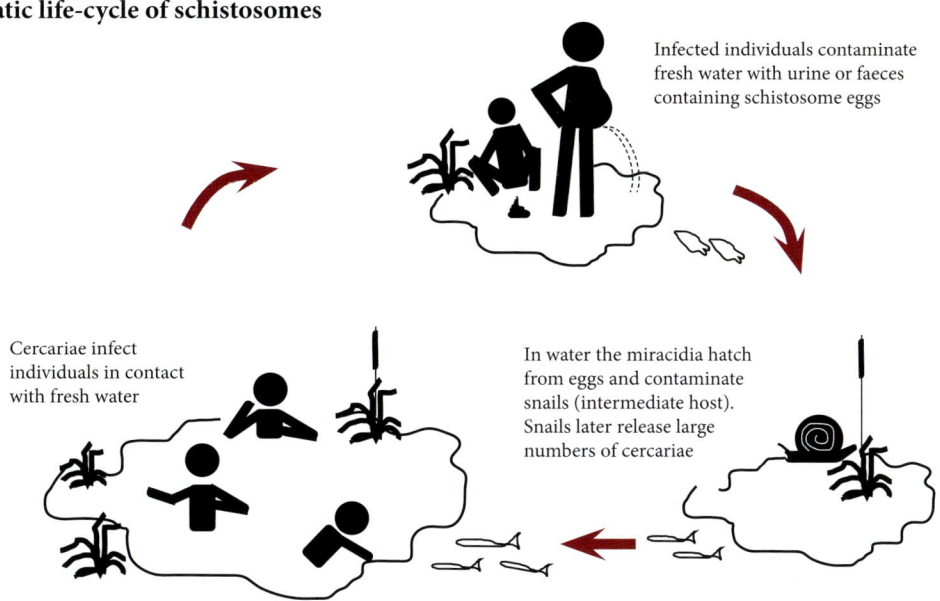

Infected individuals contaminate fresh water with urine or faeces containing schistosome eggs

Cercariae infect individuals in contact with fresh water

In water the miracidia hatch from eggs and contaminate snails (intermediate host). Snails later release large numbers of cercariae

Table 1.3 Effects of schistosomiasis and soil-transmitted helminth infections in humans

Effect	Sign of morbidity	Parasite	Reference
Nutritional impairment	Intestinal bleeding, impaired iron status, anaemia	Hookworms *S. mansoni*	Stoltzfus et al., 1996 Friedman et al., 2005 Hall et al., 2008
	Urinary tract bleeding (haematuria), impaired iron status, anaemia	*S. haematobium*	Farid, 1993
	Malabsorption of nutrients	*A. lumbricoides*	Solomons, 1993 Crompton & Nesheim, 2002
	Competition for micronutrients	*A. lumbricoides*	Curtale et al., 1993
	Impaired growth	*A. lumbricoides* *S. haematobium*	Taren et al., 1987; Stephenson et al., 2000
	Loss of appetite and reduction of food intake	*A. lumbricoides*	Stephenson et al., 1993
	Diarrhoea or dysentery	*T. trichiura* *S. mansoni*	Callender et al., 1998 Lambertucci, 1993
Cognitive impairment	Reduction in fluency and memory	*T. trichiura* *A. lumbricoides* Hookworms *S. haematobium*	Nokes et al., 1992 Kvalsvig et al., 1991 Jukes et al., 2002
Conditions requiring surgical intervention	Intestinal obstruction	*A. lumbricoides*	de Silva et al., 1997
	Rectal prolapse	*T. trichiura*	WHO, 1981
Tissue reactions	Granuloma reactions to eggs in the mucosa of the urogenital system, intestine and in the liver	*S. haematobium,* *S. mansoni,* *S. japonicum*	Gryseels et al., 2006
	Obstructive uropathy, calcified bladder, cancer of the bladder	*S. haematobium*	Vennervald & Dunne, 2004
	Fibrosis of the portal tracts, hepatomegaly, ascites	*S. mansoni*	Lambertucci, 1993

Background

A mathematical method has recently been developed (de Silva & Hall, 2010) for estimating the combined prevalence of STH infections based on knowing the prevalence of any one STH infection (*A. lumbricoides*, *T. trichiura* and hookworm) presented separately (see *section 2.3*).

Prevalence is the key indicator for the initial selection of the control measures for schistosomiasis and STH infections (see Chapter 2 on planning). This basic information is normally available in each country (WHO/NTD country profiles are available online; the web link is given in *Annex 1*), and allows countries to start planning control activities without the need to collect further epidemiological data.

B. *Intensity of infection* is a measure of the number of worms infecting an individual or a community. It can be measured indirectly by counting the number of parasite eggs in a small volume of faeces or urine.

The numbers of worms per person are not distributed evenly in the infected population. Most individuals will have infections of light or moderate intensity, while a few will have infections of heavy intensity. Heavily infected individuals suffer most of the clinical consequences and are the major source of infection for the rest of the community. The proportion of heavily infected individuals is therefore a particularly important indicator for monitoring the impact of interventions (see *section 4.5*).

1.5 Purpose of the control programme

The only definitive solution for eliminating schistosomiasis and STH infections is improvement in environmental conditions and a change in risk behaviours. Without these improvements, the prevalence of infection will tend to return to original pre-treatment levels within a few months of a round of deworming. The deworming intervention must therefore be repeated periodically.

Despite reinfection, important benefits are always achieved by periodic drug treatment. These include:

- reducing the number of heavily infected people;
- reducing environmental contamination and risk of infection for other people;
- reducing micronutrient loss (e.g. iron loss through intestinal bleeding in hookworm infection);
- improving nutritional status;
- reducing the lesions of the urinary tract and the liver.
- improving cognitive functions, learning abilities.

1.6 School-age children are the major targets for deworming programmes

More than 610 million children of school age are at risk of morbidity due to schistosomiasis or soil-transmitted helminthiases (WHO, 2011). School-age children are an important high-risk group for schistosomiasis and STH infections because the infections occur:

- during a period of intense physical growth and rapid metabolism resulting in increased nutritional needs; when these needs are not adequately met, growth is impaired and children are more susceptible to infection;
- during a period of intense learning; when children are infected, learning capacities are significantly diminished;
- in a setting of continuous exposure to contaminated soil and water; children generally lack awareness of the need for good personal hygiene and like to play with soil and water.

Regular deworming reduces both the morbidity caused by these infections and the occurrence of severe complications. Treatment of school-age children through schools is efficient: use of the school infrastructure reduces distribution costs and provides the opportunity to reach both enrolled and non-enrolled school-age children (see *section 3.5*).

The purpose of control programmes is to reduce worm loads and keep them low. Children will become re-infected, but repeated treatment will ensure that, most of the time, they will have few worms, and this will improve their chances of growing and learning.

The benefits of a school-based control programme can also be extended to other high-risk groups (that is, preschool children and pregnant women) and to the community at large: treatment of infected children reduces the number of helminth eggs and larvae reaching the environment and so reduces the risk of infection for other people in the community.

WHO has set a target of regular delivery of anthelminthic treatment to at least 75% of school-age children in endemic areas.

1.7 Components of a helminth control programme

A school-based control programme comprising deworming, improvement of water and sanitation, and health education can reduce the transmission of schistosomiasis and STH infections and prevent the development of associated morbidity.

A comprehensive control programme should include all three of these components. When intensity of infection is high, regular drug treatment should be considered as a first-line rapid control measure. Improved water and sanitation and health education components should be implemented according to the epidemiological situation and the resources available.

1.7.1 Periodic drug treatment

Periodic drug treatment – deworming – *reduces morbidity* by reducing the worm burden. The immediate outcome is a rapid improvement in child health as well as, in the case of schistosomiasis, a reduction in the risk of developing irreversible pathology in adulthood.

The drugs used to treat the most common schistosome and STH infections are effective, inexpensive and easy to administer. They have been through extensive safety testing and have been used in millions of individuals with few and minor side-effects. Recommended treatments for use in public health interventions are summarized in *Table 1.4*.

Albendazole and mebendazole have very similar modes of action and very similar efficacies (measured as egg reduction rate – ERR) after a single administration (Keiser and Utzinger, 2008):

- both drugs are highly efficacious for *A. lumbricoides* (ERR range for albendazole, 95–100%; ERR range for mebendazole, 96–99%);
- mebendazole is slightly more efficacious for *T. trichiura* (ERR range for albendazole, 53–89%; ERR range for mebendazole, 81–90%);
- albendazole is slightly more efficacious for hookworms (ERR range for albendazole, 64–100%; ERR range for mebendazole, 52–100%).

When deworming is administered regularly over a few years, the results obtained with either of the two drugs are optimal for all the STH species (see effect of mebendazole on hookworm in Cambodia; Sinuon et al., 2007) or albendazole for *T. trichiura* in Mexico (Flisser et al., 2008).

For US$ 2, it is possible to procure STH treatment for 100 children. For US$ 2, it is possible to procure schistosomiasis treatment for 10 children.

Several drug donation programmes are in place to support endemic countries (see *Annex 1*).

The cost of drug distribution (including training, monitoring, transport) in a school-based programme is extremely low. A recent study (Montresor et al., 2010) estimated the average cost to be between US$ 0.03 (when only STH are addressed) and US$ 0.13 (when also schistosomiasis is covered) per child.

Table 1.4 Drugs recommended for use in large-scale school deworming programmes[a]

	Drugs	Dose	Approx. cost per dose (US$)
Schistosomes	praziquantel (600 mg)	40 mg/kg	0.20[b]
Soil-transmitted helminths[c]	albendazole (400 mg) or	400 mg[d]	0.02
	mebendazolee (500 mg)[e] or	500 mg[d]	0.02
	levamisole	80 mg[d]	0.01

[a] WHO, 2002.
[b] The praziquantel dose varies between 1 and 4 tablets: on average, 2.5 tablets are necessary to treat a school-age child. The cost of each tablet is approximately US$ 0.08.
[c] Pyrantel pamoate (10 mg/kg) is also among the WHO-recommended drugs for the treatment of STH infections but is not commonly used for large-scale school deworming programmes because the dosing is based on weight, which is not easily measured in endemic settings. The combination pyrantel–oxantel has been proposed as a valuable alternative to mebendazole and albendazole (Albonico et al., 2002) but is not yet widely used.
[d] Same dose for all school-age children.
[e] *The International pharmacopoeia* (WHO, 2010a) recently recognized that one of the mebendazole polymorphs (mebendazole exists in three polymorphs A, B and C) is significantly more active than the others. When procuring mebendazole, programme managers are therefore advised to select mebendazole with a high level of polymorph C.

Figure 1.6 Main activities of a deworming programme for school-age children

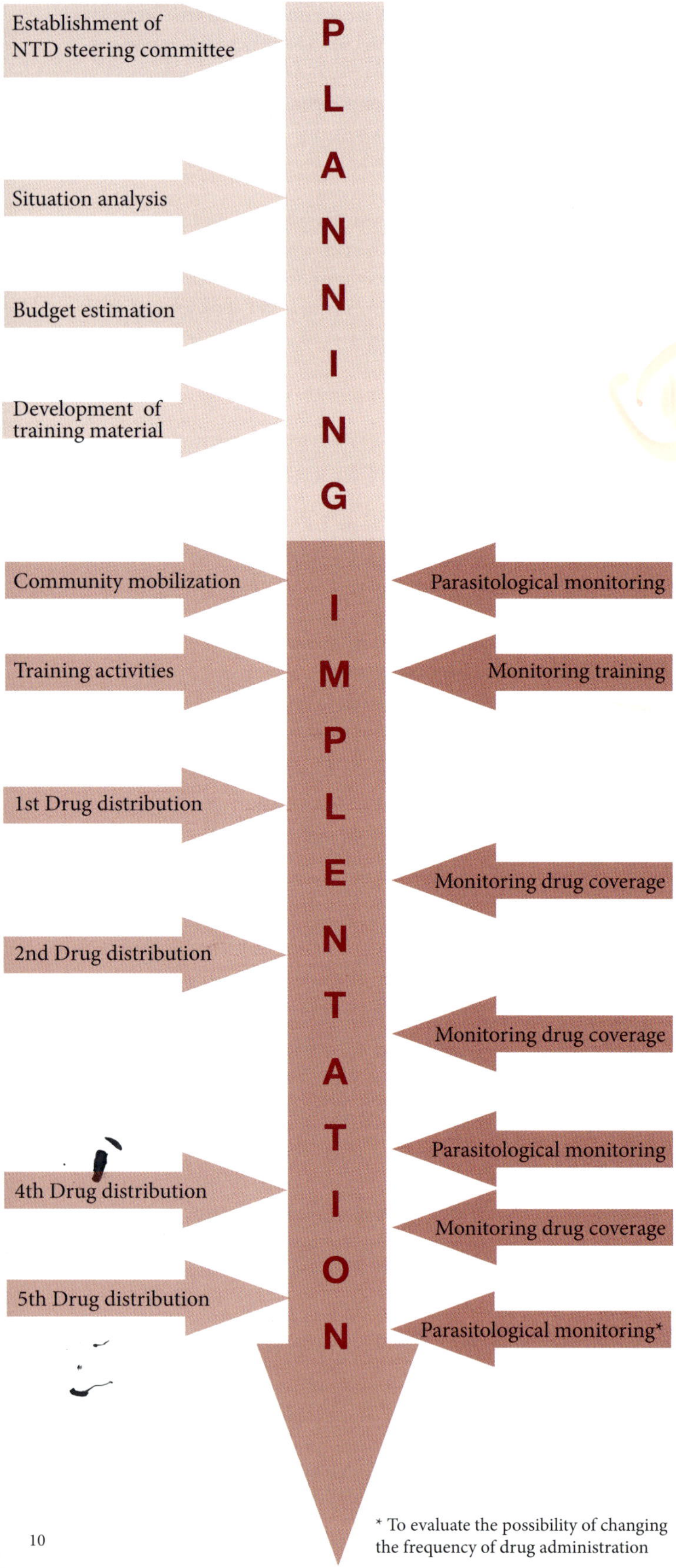

Establishment of NTD steering committee

Situation analysis

Budget estimation

Development of training material

PLANNING

Community mobilization

Parasitological monitoring

Training activities

Monitoring training

IMPLEMENTATION

1st Drug distribution

Monitoring drug coverage

2nd Drug distribution

Monitoring drug coverage

Parasitological monitoring

4th Drug distribution

Monitoring drug coverage

5th Drug distribution

Parasitological monitoring*

* To evaluate the possibility of changing the frequency of drug administration

1.7.2 Clean water and sanitation facilities

Provision of clean water and improved sanitation decreases the *transmission* of infection by reducing contact with soil and/or water contaminated by helminth eggs.

Coupled with behavioural changes, better sanitation and water supply are long-term measures that sustain the health improvements of schoolchildren.

Schools, particularly those in rural areas, often lack clean drinking-water and adequate sanitation facilities. Guidelines on improving sanitation to acceptable levels in schools with limited financial resources have recently been developed (UNICEF/WHO, 2009).

1.7.3 Health and hygiene education

Health and hygiene education reduces *transmission* and *reinfection* by encouraging healthy behaviours.

Increasing children's awareness of the problem and extending community involvement are important elements of a deworming programme targeting school-age children. WHO has published a document indicating the health education priorities that should be addressed in schools to reduce schistosomiasis and STH infections and sustain health benefits (WHO, 1996).

1.8 Steps for implementing a helminth control programme in schools

Using a schematic timeline, *Figure 1.6* illustrates the main activities to be considered when planning a helminth control programme for the school-age population.

These activities can be classified into three groups: planning, implementation and monitoring activities; and are discussed in detail in Chapters 2, 3 and 4.

1.9 Cost-effectiveness, sustainability and integration

School-based control of schistosomiasis and soil-transmitted helminthiases ranks as one of the most cost-effective public health interventions, with an average cost per DALY averted (US$ 14) similar to that of immunization programmes for the vaccine-preventable diseases of childhood (US$ 10–20 per DALY averted; Laxminarayan et al., 2006). In a study conducted in Cambodia, in which a schistosomiasis control programme was analysed from an economic standpoint, it was estimated that, for each dollar invested in schistosomiasis control, the return exceeded US$ 3.80 in increased productivity (Croce et al., 2010). Such positive outcomes are the result of the extremely low cost of the drug and the use of the existing school infrastructure and personnel for programme delivery. Success, however, depends on the political will and commitment of the government concerned.

Further cost reductions and improved efficiency can be achieved by integrating school deworming with other interventions (see *section 3.6* for details).

The treatment of schistosomiasis and STH infections in school-age children should be harmonized with other large-scale drug interventions taking place in the community (WHO, 2006). For example, where albendazole is distributed annually to an entire community as part of lymphatic filariasis control, it is important to allow an interval of approximately 6 months before the distribution of albendazole in schools in order to have the maximum effect (see also *section 2.5*).

WHO is supporting ministries of health in endemic countries to prepare integrated plans for NTD control that include a school deworming component.

1.10   Key stakeholders in school-based deworming programmes

Central government involvement is crucial, particularly in developing and adopting a national policy on helminth control. Programme managers therefore have a responsibility to ensure that the potential impact of programmes is made known to different government sectors. Health ministries should be aware of the opportunity provided by schools in furthering their goals of promoting health; ministries of education should be aware that helminth control will increase the learning potential and academic achievements of the children.

The school system is critical to sustainability. Every year, thousands of teachers in endemic countries take a leading role in administering deworming drugs and providing health education messages to school-age children. By including health education on personal hygiene and on prevention of worm infections in school curricula and by raising sanitation standards in school in partnership with other sectors, the school system can contribute substantially to the improvement of the health of schoolchildren.

Children's parents, families and communities also play an essential role. With the active backing of other advocates (for example, ministries of health and education,

nongovernmental organizations), families furnish substantial support for school-based programmes. They can provide practical assistance, such as helping with the logistics during deworming days and with dissemination of health education messages, and can also facilitate the participation of non-enrolled school-age children in the deworming campaigns. The involvement of families, with clear communication of the reasons for, and objectives of, the intervention would counter any perception that children are forced to take medicines that are unsafe or for reasons other than protection of their health.

1.11   Partnering for the control of neglected tropical diseases

Collaboration among different departments of the ministry of health (for example, managers responsible for the control of schistosomiasis and STH infections, onchocerciasis and lymphatic filariasis, and managers responsible for vaccination activities), other ministries (such as education) and other local partners (nongovernmental organizations, academia, parents' associations, teacher associations, private companies) is essential for the efficient implementation not only of the deworming of schoolchildren but also of NTD control in general (see also *section 2.1*). International partnerships – for example with other governments, international organizations, nongovernmental organizations and donor agencies – can be explored as a means of supporting control activities (see *Annex 1*).

1.12   Deworming school-age children and the Millennium Development Goals

Experience from several countries has produced solid evidence that periodic treatment of school-age children is a strategy with enormous potential for development (Molyneux et al., 2005). Periodic deworming of school-age children provides an important contribution to the achievement of four of the Millennium Development Goals (WHO, 2010b):

Goal 1 – Eradicate extreme poverty and hunger
Deworming boosts the prospects of school-age children earning their way out of poverty. The improvements in intellectual development and cognition that follow deworming appear to have a substantial impact on professional income later in life (Miguel & Kremer, 2001).

Goal 2 – Achieve universal primary education
In developing countries, treatment of school-age children with deworming drugs can reduce primary school absenteeism by 25% (United States Government, 2003) and improve learning capacities (Nokes et al., 1992).

Goal 3 – Promote gender equality and empower women

A girl's best start in life is a good education. Education also provides her best chance of finding employment. Although the gender gap in education is slowly closing in developing countries, there are still more boys than girls in schools. Deworming programmes, especially when associated with other measures such as school meals and take-home rations, have been shown to contribute to increased school enrolment and retention rates of girls (Khanal & Walgate, 2002).

Goal 6 – Combat HIV/AIDS, malaria and other diseases

While helminth infections do not cause the same high mortality as AIDS and malaria, the morbidity and disability that they cause can significantly impair the health status, physical and mental development, and productivity of huge numbers of poor people. Reducing schistosomiasis and STH infections builds the very foundation of good health. Evidence is starting to emerge that helminth infections may actually influence the clinical burden of AIDS (Fincham et al., 2003) and malaria (Kirwan et al., 2010). Moreover, recent studies indicate that worm infections may disrupt the immune response in ways that could speed up the progression from HIV infection to AIDS (Erikstrup et al., 2008).

References

Albonico M et al. (2002). Evaluation of the efficacy of pyrantel–oxantel for the treatment of soil-transmitted nematode infections. *Transactions of the Royal Society of Tropical Medicine and Hygiene*, 96:685–690.

Brito LL et al. (2006). Moderate- and low-intensity co-infections by intestinal helminths and *Schistosoma mansoni*, dietary iron intake, and anemia in Brazilian children. *American Journal of Tropical Medicine and Hygiene*, 75:939–944.

Callender JE et al. (1998). Growth and development four years after treatment for the *Trichuris* dysentery syndrome. *Acta Paediatrica*, 87:1247–1249.

Croce D et al. (2010) Cost-effectiveness of a successful schistosomiasis control programme in Cambodia (1995–2006). *Acta Tropica*, 113:279–284.

Crompton DWT, Nesheim MC (2002). Nutritional impact of intestinal helminthiasis during the human life cycle. *Annual Review of Nutrition*, 22:35–59.

Curtale F et al. (1993). Intestinal helminths and risk of anaemia among Nepalese children. *Panminerva Medica*, 35:159–166.

de Silva N, Hall A (2010). Using the prevalence of individual species of intestinal nematode worms to estimate the combined prevalence of any species. *PLoS Neglected Tropical Diseases*, 4:e655.

de Silva NR, Chan MS, Bundy DA (1997). Morbidity and mortality due to ascariasis: re-estimation and sensitivity analysis of global numbers at risk. *Tropical Medicine & International Health*, 2:519–528.

de Silva NR et al. (2003). Soil-transmitted helminth infections: updating the global picture. *Trends in Parasitology*, 19:547–551.

Erikstrup C et al. (2008). Schistosomiasis and infection with human immunodeficiency virus 1 in rural Zimbabwe: systemic inflammation during co-infection and after treatment for schistosomiasis. *American Journal of Tropical Medicine and Hygiene*, 79:331–337.

Farid Z (1993). Schistosomes with terminal-spined eggs: pathological and clinical aspects. In: Jordan P et al., eds. *Human schistosomiasis*. Wallingford, England, CAB International.

Fincham JE, Markus MB, Adams VJ (2003). Could control of soil-transmitted helminthic infection influence the HIV/AIDS pandemic? *Acta Tropica*, 86:315–333.

Flisser A et al. (2008). Using national health weeks to deliver deworming to children: lessons from Mexico. *Journal of Epidemiology and Community Health*, 62:314-317.

Friedman JF, Kanzaria HK, McGarvey ST (2005). Human schistosomiasis and anemia: the relationship and potential mechanisms. *Trends in Parasitology*, 21:386–392.

Gryseels B et al. (2006). *Human schistosomiasis*. Lancet, 368:1106–1118.

Hall A, Hewitt G, Tuffrey V, & de Silva N (2008) A review and meta-analysis of the impact of intestinal worms on child growth and nutrition. *Maternal and Child Nutrition*, 4(Suppl. 1):118–236.

Hotez PJ et al. (2009). Rescuing the bottom billion through control of neglected tropical diseases. *Lancet*, 373:1570–1575.

Jukes MC et al. (2002). Heavy schistosomiasis associated with poor short-term memory and slower reaction times in Tanzanian schoolchildren. *Tropical Medicine & International Health*, 7:104–117.

Keiser J et al. (2002). Association between *Schistosoma mansoni* and hookworm infections among schoolchildren in Côte d'Ivoire. *Acta Tropica*, 84:31–41.

Keiser J, Utzinger J. (2008). Efficacy of current drugs against soil-transmitted helminth infections: systematic review and meta-analysis. *Journal of the American Medical Association*, 299:1937–1948.

Khanal P, Walgate R (2002). Nepal deworming programme ready to go worldwide. *Bulletin of the World Health Organization*, 80:423–424.

Kirwan P et al. (2010). Impact of repeated four-monthly anthelmintic treatment on *Plasmodium* infection in preschool children: a double-blind placebo-controlled randomized trial. *BMC Infectious Diseases*, 10:277.

Kvalsvig JD, Cooppan RM, Connolly KJ (1991). The effects of parasite infections on cognitive processes in children. *Annals of Tropical Medicine and Parasitology*, 85:551–568.

Lambertucci R (1993). *Schistosoma mansoni*: pathological and clinical aspects. In: Jordan P et al., eds. *Human schistosomiasis*. Wallingford, England, CAB International.

Laxminarayan R et al. (2006). Advancement of global health: key messages from the Disease Control Priorities Project. *Lancet*, 367:1193–1208.

Miguel E, Kremer M (2001). *Worms: education and health externalities in Kenya*. Cambridge, MA, National Bureau of Economic Research (NBER Working Paper No. 8481).

Molyneux DH, Hotez PJ, Fenwick A (2005). "Rapid-impact interventions": how a policy of integrated control for Africa's neglected tropical diseases could benefit the poor. *PLoS Medicine*, 2:e336.

Montresor A et al. (2010). Estimation of the cost of large-scale school deworming programmes with benzimidazoles. *Transactions of the Royal Society of Tropical Medicine and Hygiene*, 104:129–132.

Nokes C et al. (1992). Parasitic helminth infection and cognitive function in school children. *Proceedings of the Royal Society of London B*, 247:77–81.

Pullan R, Brooker S (2008). The health impact of polyparasitism in humans: are we under-estimating the burden of parasitic diseases? *Parasitology*, 135:783–794.

Sinuon M et al. (2007). Control of Schistosoma mekongi in Cambodia: results of eight years of control activities in the two endemic provinces. *Transactions of the Royal Society of Tropical Medicine and Hygiene*, 101:34–39.

Solomons NW (1993). Pathways to the impairment of human nutritional status by gastrointestinal pathogens. *Parasitology*, 107(Suppl.):S19–S35.

Stephenson LS, Latham MC, Ottesen EA (2000). Malnutrition and parasitic helminth infections. *Parasitology*, 121(Suppl.):S23–S38.

Stephenson LS et al. (1993). Physical fitness, growth and appetite of Kenyan school boys with hookworm, *Trichuris trichiura* and *Ascaris lumbricoides* infections are improved four months after a single dose of albendazole. *Journal of Nutrition*, 123:1036–1046.

Stoltzfus RJ et al. (1996). Hemoquant determination of hookworm-related blood loss and its role in iron deficiency in African children. *American Journal of Tropical Medicine and Hygiene*, 55:399–404.

Taren DL et al. (1987). Contributions of ascariasis to poor nutritional status in children from Chiriqui Province, Republic of Panama. *Parasitology*, 95:603–613.

UNICEF/WHO (2009). *Water, sanitation and hygiene standards for schools in low-cost settings*. Geneva, World Health Organization.

United States Government (2003). *The Annual Report of the Council of Economic Advisers*. Washington, DC, United States Printing Office:241.

Vennervald BJ, Dunne DW (2004). Morbidity in schistosomiasis: an update. *Current Opinion in Infectious Diseases*, 17:439–447.

WHO (1981). *Intestinal protozoan and helminthic infections. Report of a WHO Scientific Group*. Geneva, World Health Organization (WHO Technical Report Series, No. 666).

WHO (1996). *Report of the WHO Informal Consultation on the use of chemotherapy for the control of morbidity due to soil-transmitted nematodes in humans*, Geneva, 29 April to 1 May 1996. Geneva, World Health Organization (WHO/CTD/SIP/96.2).

WHO (2002). *Prevention and control of schistosomiasis and soil-transmitted helminthiasis*. Report of a WHO Expert Committee. Geneva, World Health Organization (WHO Technical Report Series, No. 912).

WHO (2006). *Preventive chemotherapy in human helminthiasis. Coordinated use of anthelminthic drugs in control interventions: a manual for health professionals and programme managers*. Geneva, World Health Organization.

WHO (2010a). *International pharmacopeia*. Geneva, World Health Organization.

WHO (2010b). *Working to overcome the global impact of neglected tropical diseases: first WHO report on neglected tropical diseases*. Geneva, World Health Organization (WHO/HTM/NTD/2010.1).

WHO (2011). Soil-transmitted helminthiases: estimates of the number of children needing preventive chemotherapy and number treated, 2009. *Weekly Epidemiological Record*, 86:257–266.

PLANNING

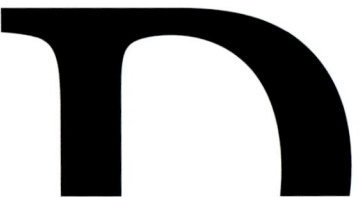

Deworming school-age children should be conceived as a part of a larger national strategy for the integrated control and elimination of NTDs. Deworming activities should therefore be planned, implemented and monitored in coordination with other NTD control activities.

Photograph by WHO

2.1 Establishing a steering committee for the integrated control of neglected tropical diseases

Deworming school-age children should be conceived as a part of a larger national strategy for the integrated control and elimination of NTDs. Deworming activities should therefore be planned, implemented and monitored in coordination with other NTD control activities (WHO 2006).

WHO encourages endemic countries to establish a coordination mechanism – the NTD steering committee – with representation from various departments of the relevant ministries (for example, from the ministry of health: managers responsible for the control and elimination of STH, schistosomiasis, onchocerciasis, lymphatic filariasis and vaccine-preventable diseases; from the ministry of education: school health department) and from other agencies (international and nongovernmental organizations, research institutions). This allows all the partners working for NTD control to have a clear picture of what the others are doing, or can do, and provides in-depth knowledge of local

resources that are potentially available for implementation of the programme.

2.2 Situation analysis

The first step in the successful development of an integrated plan for NTD control (including deworming of school-age children) is a situation analysis to provide the NTD steering committee with an in-depth understanding of the epidemiological status of relevant NTDs and of current NTD control activities in the country.

The situation analysis should start with a review of available data to help define the context for exploratory meetings with decision-makers, communities and potential donors. If adequate resources are available, the analysis can be detailed and comprehensive, but the most appropriate initial approach is usually the collection of available data that can be achieved at relatively low cost. Information to be collected during the situation analysis is suggested in *Table 2.1*.

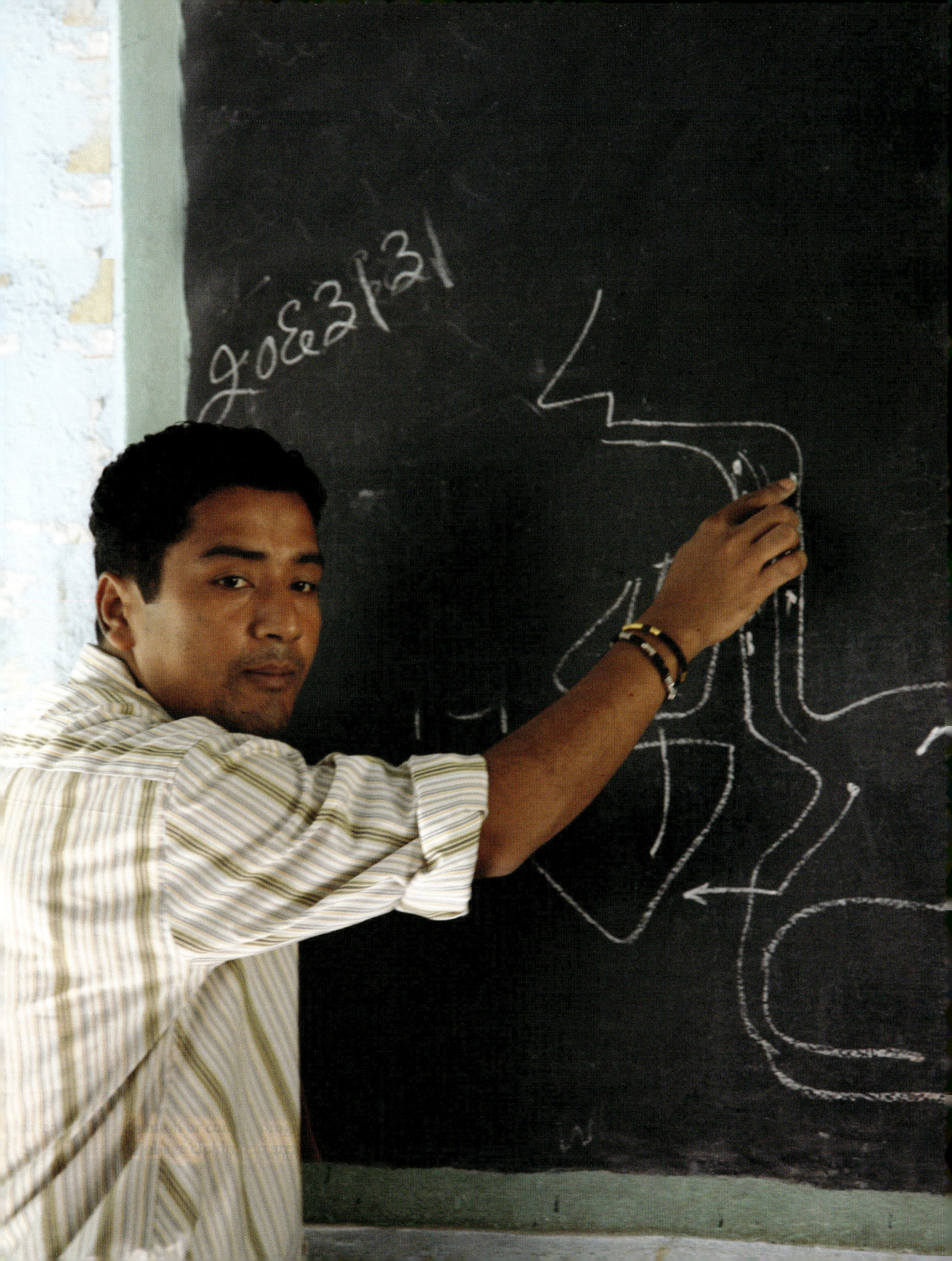

2.3 Baseline epidemiological data

Baseline epidemiological information is essential:

- to define the areas of the country where different interventions are needed;
- to estimate drug requirements;
- to select appropriate control measures;
- to determine the frequency of interventions.

Organizing a survey to collect parasitological data can require substantial financial and human resources, and may cause significant delays in the application of urgent control measures. Whenever possible, therefore, existing epidemiological data, including historical records, should be used to save time and resources.

Epidemiological data could be obtained locally from ministry of health files (unpublished surveys), from research institutions (theses or publications) and from the periodic reports submitted by health units.

Significant resources have recently been invested in collecting baseline epidemiological data on schistosomiasis and STH infections in several countries, and these data have been made available through web sites (links are provided in *Annex 1*):

Table 2.1 Data needed for a situation analysis

Data to be collected	Suggested sources	Use	Comments
Epidemiological data • Prevalence of schistosomiasis and STH by ecological zone	MoH, publications, theses, hospital records, previous surveys, NGOs	• Determination of intervention areas • Selection of control strategy • To serve as baseline	Maps are available on line (see *Annex 1*)
School data • Size of school-age population • Number of schools and teachers by district, province and ecological zone • School enrolment rate	Census data, population estimates, MoE (e.g. education management information system)	• Determination of programme size • Evaluation of the extent of non-enrolment	WHO databank provides this information (see *Annex 1*)
Control activities data • Current experience with school deworming conducted by MoH, MoE, NGOs • Ongoing mass drug administration through the Programme for the Elimination of Lymphatic Filariasis[a]	MoH, MoE, NGOs MoH, MoE, NGOs	• To avoid duplication • Assessment of the capacity of national authorities • Maximizing the use of available resources	WHO databank provides this information (see *Annex 1*)
Logistic opportunities • Possible ways to dispatch drugs to districts and schools • Possible ways to gather teachers for training	MoH or MoE, NGOs	• Reducing costs • Maximizing the use of available resources	
Existence of health education resources • Training and health education materials available or in use in schools, dispensaries, etc.	MoH, MoE, NGOs	• Maximizing the use of available health education materials.	Link to examples of health education are provided in *Annex 1*
Opportunities for social mobilization • Information about the possibility of developing and broadcasting television and radio advertisements	National television and radio	• Evaluating the costs of a media campaign in support of the deworming intervention	

[a] Albendazole is distributed annually to the entire population in areas endemic for lymphatic filariasis in the context of the Global Programme for the Elimination of Lymphatic Filariasis. This intervention has an impact also on the epidemiology of STH.

MoE = ministry of education; MoH = ministry of health; NGO = nongovernmental organization; NTD = neglected tropical disease; SCH = schistosomiasis; STH = soil-transmitted helminthiases.

- Extensive data on schistosomiasis are presented in the Atlas of the global distribution of schistosomiasis (WHO/CEGET, 1987).
- For Africa, information on STH infections is available from the Global Atlas of Helminth Infections.
- Data on schistosomiasis and STH infections for each endemic country are available in WHO country profiles; these are periodically updated and indicate areas where data are insufficient and additional surveys should be conducted.

In most cases, the available data for a country are sufficient to allow appropriate schistosomiasis and STH control activities to be established.

The following assumptions should be made for the appropriate use of the available epidemiological data in order to maximize the resources available for control:

- Where no control activities have been implemented, even 10–15-year-old data can provide a clear indication of the epidemiological situation.
- In homogeneous ecological zones, the prevalence of schistosomiasis and STH infections are also assumed to be homogeneous.
- Homogeneous ecological zones of STH and SCH vary in size:

  - In the case of STH, since the infections have a wide geographical distribution, each zone normally covers several districts in a country.
  - In the case of SCH, since the disease is focally transmitted around water bodies, the limit of ecological zones can be within the district (for example, coastal and interior areas). The main areas endemic for schistosomiasis are normally known in each country (see WHO/NTD country profiles); however, it may be necessary to collect data in sentinel sites during the implementation phase (see *Chapter 5*) in order to refine information on the number of schools to be targeted for treatment.

- Wherever schistosomes are transmitted, it is likely that STHs are also endemic (Yajima et al., 2011); consequently, every time praziquantel is distributed, the distribution of albendazole or mebendazole is also justified.

The aim of the analysis of epidemiological data is to classify communities according to their risk for developing morbidity due to schistosomiasis and STH infections and to define the type of control intervention needed.

The suggested indicator for guiding decisions on the control of schistosomiasis and STH infections is the prevalence of infection. This indicator, normally available from previous surveys conducted in the zone, is used to decide whether helminth infections are a health problem in schools and communities.

In the case of STH, it is important to use the prevalence of any STH infection (see *section 1.4*).

Frequently, the prevalence of each parasite infection is recorded separately. A mathematical method for estimating the prevalence of any STH infection from the prevalence of single STH infections has been described by de Silva & Hall (2010).

The prevalence of any STH infection (P_{ath}) can be estimated using the following equation:

$$P_{ath} = \frac{(a + t + h) - (a \times t + a \times h + t \times h) + (a \times t \times h)}{1.06}$$

where

a = prevalence of ascariasis (expressed as a proportion)
t = prevalence of trichuriasis (expressed as a proportion)
h = prevalence of hookworm infection (expressed as a proportion)

For example in the case in which
the prevalence of ascariasis is 50% (a = 0.50)
the prevalence of trichuriasis is 40% (t = 0.40)
the prevalence of hookworm infection is 30% (h = 0.30)

the prevalence of any STH infection estimated with the equation is 75% (P_{ath} = 0.75).

2.3.1   School questionnaires for urinary schistosomiasis

WHO has developed a method for ranking schools in order of need of intervention in areas endemic for urinary schistosomiasis. The method relies on the fact that visible haematuria (blood in the urine) is an indicator of a heavy infection that can be easily recognized by the children. The method requires the distribution to each school of short questionnaires asking children whether they have seen blood in their urine at any time during the past month. This method:

- provides indirect evidence of the extent of urinary schistosomiasis in a school;
- enables schools to be ranked in order of severity of schistosomiasis;
- informs the setting of priorities for treatment, where funds are limited.

Detailed procedures for using the questionnaire approach are discussed in *The schistosomiasis manual* (Chitsulo et al., 1995).

2.3.2 Selection of control measures

Baseline epidemiological data should be used to classify the areas where schools are placed into categories, as shown in *Table 2.2* for schistosomiasis and *Table 2.3* for STH infections.

This classification provides an indication of the need and frequency of drug administration in the school-age population and the urgency of other measures, such as health education activities and improvement in sanitation and water supply.

If epidemiological data are collected after years of control activities, different thresholds are suggested (see *section 2.5*).

It should be noted that the laboratory techniques used to collect parasitological data may miss some light infections and therefore the prevalence measured may be somewhat lower than the "real" prevalence in the community (Booth

Table 2.2 Recommended control strategies for schistosomiasis in school-age children

Category	Prevalence of schistosomiasis among school-age children at baseline	Control strategy	
		Preventive chemotherapy	Additional interventions
Schools in high-risk areas	≥50% if based on parasitological methods *or* ≥30% if based on questionnaires for visible haematuria	Treat all school-age children (enrolled and non-enrolled) once a year	Improve sanitation and water supply Provide health education
Schools in moderate-risk areas	≥10% and <50% if based on parasitological methods or >1% and <30% if based on questionnaires for visible haematuria	Treat all school-age children (enrolled and non-enrolled) once every two years	Improve sanitation and water supply Provide health education
Schools in low-risk areas	≥1% and <10% if based on parasitological methods	Treat all school-age children (enrolled and non-enrolled) twice during their primary-school years (e.g. once on entry and once on exit)	Improve sanitation and water supply Provide health education

Table 2.3 Recommended control strategies for soil-transmitted helminth (STH) infections in school-age children[a]

Category	Prevalence of any STH infection at baseline	Control strategy	
		Preventive chemotherapy	Additional interventions
Schools in high-risk areas	≥50%	Treat all school-age children (enrolled and non-enrolled) twice a year[b]	Improve sanitation and water supply Provide health education
Schools in low-risk areas	≥20% and <50%	Treat all school-age children (enrolled and non-enrolled) once a year	Improve sanitation and water supply Provide health education

[a] When the prevalence of any STH infection is under 20%, large-scale preventive chemotherapy interventions are not recommended. Affected individuals should be treated on a case-by-case basis.

[b] If the resources are available and the prevalence is towards the higher end of the interval, a third drug distribution might be added (in this case, the frequency will be every 4 months).

et al., 2003). This fact was taken into consideration when the thresholds for recommending the treatment strategies were established (WHO, 2006).

These thresholds are given as an indication: intuitively, there is not a big difference between 49% prevalence and 50%. According to *Table 2.3*, one treatment a year is indicated the first case and two in the second case. Flexibility in selecting control measures may be necessary, and managers of control programmes may decide to use more intensive interventions if resources are available.

2.4 School data

Knowing the number of children to be reached allows a rough calculation of the cost of the intervention: on average, for every one million children to be treated for STH infections, approximately US$ 20 000 should be budgeted for drugs (if not donated) and US$ 33 000 for other components such as training, distribution and monitoring (Montresor et al., 2010). For schistosomiasis, the costs are higher – approximately US$ 180 000 for drugs and US$ 50 000 for the other components.

Information on enrolment rates, number and size of schools, number of teachers, and the school calendar is essential for assessing whether the school system will be able to reach most children and whether alternative methods should be used to reach non-enrolled or non-attending children (see *section 3.7*).

2.5 Data from control activities for other diseases

Knowledge of current or past NTD control activities in the targeted areas is very useful for the following purposes:

- to avoid duplication of deworming activities in the same target population and thus save financial resources;
- to identify experienced NGOs or other institutions that are already trusted by the community and interested in helping with drug administration, capacity-building, programme oversight and quality control of the deworming programme;
- to identify schools where teachers have been trained for deworming in the past; this will reduce training costs because teachers are already familiar with the deworming intervention;
- to identify the presence of control programmes providing services to the school population (for example, for trachoma control), which would allow the deworming programme to use an existing infrastructure thereby significantly reducing expenditures.

A case in point is the distribution of albendazole in the context of the Global Programme for the Elimination Lymphatic Filariasis (GPELF). The programme distributes albendazole and ivermectin (or albendazole and diethylcarbamazine citrate) once a year to the entire population of the area endemic for lymphatic filariasis (LF). When the programme is implemented, the albendazole distribution can substitute for one deworming round for STH in schoolchildren. Coordination between the two interventions is necessary to ensure that they are separated by an interval of approximately 6 months.

The objectives of GPELF are usually achieved after approximately 5-6 years of intervention, at which point activities come to an end. At that time, it is useful to conduct a survey in a sentinel site (see *Chapter 5* for details) to evaluate whether continued STH control is necessary.

Annex 10 proposes suggestions on how to proceed with the control of STH according to the different levels of prevalence measured during the survey. The thresholds given are *suggestions only*, since experience is limited in this area. The same thresholds are provided to managers of STH control programmes intending to explore the possibility of changing the frequency of drug administration after 5–6 years of interventions with good coverage (*section 4.7*).

The thresholds are more restrictive than those provided in *Table 2.3*; prevalence is determined in a situation in which anthelminthic drugs (albendazole and ivermectin[3]) have been administered for 5-6 years. In this situation, even a moderate STH prevalence (of, for example, 20%) indicates that the parasites maintain transmission capacity despite intense drug pressure, and that prevalence would probably reach high levels within a short time if the drug intervention were to be interrupted.

2.6 Logistic opportunities

Obtaining information about existing infrastructure for dispatching drugs throughout the country is important. In several countries, an efficient drug delivery system is in place for hospitals and peripheral health units, consisting of a regular service of dedicated vehicles and a chain of central and peripheral medical stores. Such a system can accept responsibility for the distribution of drugs for the school-based deworming programme, since the size of the drug delivery (of albendazole/mebendazole and praziquantel) necessary for one round of treatment is relatively small (approximately 1 cubic metre for 250 000 tablets).

---

[3] Ivermectin is also reported to be active against STH (Marti et al., 1996).

Another opportunity to facilitate programme logistics is to meet with teachers during one of the regular sessions organized by the ministry of education for training or discussion purposes. These occasions can be used to offer training and health education material to teachers, thereby avoiding the need to organize separate meetings.

2.7 Health education materials

The promotion of personal hygiene measures (for example, hand-washing and use and maintenance of latrines) is important to maintain the health benefits achieved through deworming and is usually carried out by distributing posters and flyers to the schools.

The cost to the programme of developing and distributing health education materials is not always negligible. The availability of any existing relevant education material should be explored as a means of keeping costs down. Alternatively, health education messages can be included in school curricula and in school books, so that health education is provided to the schoolchildren as part of their normal education. Examples of health education materials are available through the WHO web site (see link in *Annex 1*).

2.8 Model budget

Preparation of a realistic budget is an essential part of the planning process and will determine whether there are sufficient local funds or whether external funding is required. The budget also serves as an advocacy tool both within a district, region or country and with external donor agencies.

School-based helminth control programmes are among the most cost-effective public health interventions because:

- they make use of existing educational infrastructure;
- they depend on low-cost, safe and effective drugs that are easily administered;
- they have maximum effect in reducing the morbidity of schistosomiasis and STH infections because school-age children are a high-risk group;
- they strengthen health awareness and provide an opportunity for additional health education with its resulting benefits.

A model budget is shown in *Table 2.4*. It is a checklist of items to be considered in the first year of implementation of a helminth control programme in an endemic area where praziquantel and albendazole are to be administered to the school-age population. All costs are given in United States dollars. Praziquantel and albendazole are indicated in this example, but health authorities should select the drugs to be used on the basis of their experience, community compliance, cost and availability.

This budget is based on the cost analysis of school deworming programmes conducted in seven countries in four WHO regions (Montresor et al., 2010). The costs were adjusted to the 2010 calendar year and an estimated amount was added for additional components (for example, outreach to non-enrolled children and development of training materials). The estimated average cost of treating each child twice in the first year of programme implementation is 42 US cents (US$ 0.42); this cost includes teacher training, health education materials and drug procurement.

From the second year onwards, the cost is reduced to 33 US cents (US$ 0.33) per child treated because training and development and distribution of health education materials do not need to be repeated. If the drugs are donated, the costs can be reduced to as little as 13 US cents (US$ 0.13) per child treated.

It should be remembered that the time spent by teachers, as well as by health personnel at central, provincial and district levels, who are providing this service as part of their routine work, represents a substantial economic and in-kind contribution that is non-negligible. This cost is estimated at 6 US cents (US$ 0.06) per child treated.

In the budget example of *Table 2.4*, the hypothetical area of intervention is made up of 4 regions (10 districts) with a total population of 4 500 000, including 1 million school-age children. The interventions needed are:

- Round 1: albendazole for the entire school-age population.
- Round 2: albendazole for the entire school-age population + praziquantel for half of the school-age population.

The peripheral health structure comprises 800 dispensaries/health centres; the personnel in these units are considered as participating actively in supervisory activities for the school-based deworming programme. There are approximately 3500 schools in the area.

The *advocacy and social mobilization activities* part of the budget includes production of advocacy material for printed and electronic media. In several countries, television and radio advertisements are broadcast at the time of the

Table 2.4 Model budget estimated to cover costs of the first year of a deworming programme for schistosomiasis and soil-transmitted helminth infections for 1 million school-age children

Component	Cost items	US$
Advocacy and social mobilization activities	Developing and reproducing (or broadcasting) advocacy/social mobilization material	5 000
Health education	Conceptualization/development of materials	–
	Adaptation/translation/production	17 500
	Material for outreach activities	17 500
Teacher/health worker training	National workshop	4 000
	Four regional workshops	8 000
	District workshops	64 500
	Duplication of training materials	1 500
Data collection in sentinel sites	4-wheel-drive vehicle	Available
	Vehicle maintenance	2 400
	Fuel	2 500
	Training of laboratory technicians	–
	Allowances for data collection team	1 500
	Laboratory material/microscopes	2 500
	Drugs administered during survey	600
	Data entry and analysis	–
Drug procurement, distribution, administration	Albendazole (2 million tablets)	40 000
	Praziquantel (1.25 million tablets)	100 000
	Insurance and freight charges (10%)	14 000
	Drug clearance and storage	22 500
	Packaging	17 500
	Periodic drug quality control	4 500
	Delivery to schools	Free of charge
	Administration to children	Free of charge
Supervision by health personnel	Central or regional personnel	8 000
	Health unit personnel (2 treatment days)	12 000
Outreach activities	First round of drug administration	35 000
	Second round of drug administration	35 000
Coverage monitoring	Duplication of forms	1 000
	Form distribution and collection	–
TOTAL		417 000
Total from year 2 (no need for training or health education materials)		324 500
Total from year 2 if drugs are donated		126 500

Note: The shaded areas in the table represent costs that can be avoided after the first year of intervention or in case of drug donation. The budget includes only direct costs and does not take into consideration indirect costs (such as time spent by teachers in administering the drug).

deworming campaigns both to invite school-age children to participate and to inform families about the reasons for the intervention. When air-time is provided free, or at reduced cost, by the state broadcasting service, the small sum invested in these activities is probably worthwhile; much higher rates are likely to be charged by commercial broadcasting services, in which case the cost-effectiveness of this intervention should be evaluated.

Health education costs are those incurred for:

- adaptation/translation/production of materials for children in school;
- development of specific material to reach non-enrolled children.

The *teacher/health worker training* budget includes costs for the cascade of training activities:

- One national workshop, conducted by national staff and attended by regional staff of the health and education ministries.
- Four regional workshops, conducted by regional staff and attended by district staff.
- Two or three workshops per district, conducted by district staff and attended by school and health unit personnel as follows:
  – 1 teacher per school (total: 3500 teachers); participation costs include transport (US$ 5 per participant) and per diem allowance (US$ 10 per participant), but these costs must be adapted in each country according to local standards;
  – 1 health worker per dispensary (total: 800 health workers), with participation costs similar to teachers.
- Adaptation/duplication/distribution of training materials.

These training costs can be avoided or significantly reduced after the first year of intervention.

The budget for *data collection in sentinel sites* covers:

- fuel and maintenance charges for the vehicle (a vehicle is assumed to be available for 2 weeks at no charge);
- parasitological data collection in 4 schools over 2 weeks (a team of 5 people, collecting data on 50 children/school, 2 schools/week, including transport time, allowance of US$ 20/person per day);
- laboratory material, including the purchase of 2 microscopes (see *Annex 2* for list of materials);
- drugs administered during the survey to all the children in the sentinel schools surveyed (total 10 000 children).

Laboratory technicians and data managers are assumed to be present and adequately trained, and the cost of data entry and data analysis is therefore not included. Data collection in sentinel sites is recommended every 2 years.

Estimating the number of albendazole or mebendazole tablets needed is simple since the dose is 1 tablet per child for each round of drug distribution. In the case of praziquantel, the estimation is more complex because the dose is different depending on the weight or height of each child. As a general rule, it is suggested that the estimate be based on 2½ tablets of praziquantel per child targeted.

Drug quantities have been calculated for the entire school-age population (enrolled and non-enrolled children) and include:

- albendazole (US$ 0.02 per tablet), twice a year to all school-age children (total: 2 million tablets);
- praziquantel (US$ 0.08 per tablet) yearly to 50% of the schools (average dose per child: 2½ tablets; total: 1.25 million tablets);
- insurance costs and freight charges (10% of the drug cost);
- customs clearance and drug storage, which can be very expensive if not properly planned in advance (see *section 3.3.1*);
- drug repackaging (US$ 5 per school):
- periodic quality control of drugs (see *section 3.3* for details).

The drug cost represents approximately 50% of the total cost of the intervention. However, several drug donation initiatives for benzimidazoles (albendazole and mebendazole) and praziquantel are available to managers of control programmes in endemic countries; total costs would be significantly reduced if drugs were donated. A list of the major drug donation initiatives and web links is given in *Annex 1*.

Supervision by health personnel of drug administration on treatment days is considered to be within the regular activities of these individuals and only minor allowances are considered to cover transport expenditure (estimated at approximately US$ 15/day).

Outreach activities for non-enrolled school-age children and information sessions for community groups are normally organized by the schools. The budget covers:

- US$ 10 per school for each drug administration round to cover the time spent by the school on activities directed to non-enrolled children.

Monitoring activities are an integral part of the programme from the outset and are budgeted for:

- duplication of forms.

Distribution and collection of forms should be organized to coincide with other programme activities and should incur no cost.

References

Booth M et al. (2003). The influence of sampling effort and the performance of the Kato-Katz technique in diagnosing *Schistosoma mansoni* and hookworm co-infections in rural Côte d'Ivoire. *Parasitology*, 127:525–531.

Chitsulo L, Lengeler C, Jenkins J (1995). *The schistosomiasis manual: a guide for the rapid identification of communities with a high prevalence of urinary schistosomiasis.* Geneva, World Health Organization (TDR/SER/MSR/95.2).

de Silva N, Hall A (2010). Using the prevalence of individual species of intestinal nematode worms to estimate the combined prevalence of any species. *PLoS Neglected Tropical Diseases*, 4:e655.

Marti H et al. (1996). A comparative trial of a single-dose ivermectin versus three days of albendazole for treatment of *Strongyloides stercoralis* and other soil-transmitted helminth infections in children. *American Journal of Tropical Medicine and Hygiene*, 55:477–481.

Montresor A et al. (2010). Estimation of the cost of large-scale school deworming programmes with benzimidazoles. *Transactions of the Royal Society of Tropical Medicine and Hygiene*, 104:129–132.

WHO (2006). *Preventive chemotherapy in human helminthiasis. Coordinated use of anthelminthic drugs in control interventions: a manual for health professionals and programme managers.* Geneva, World Health Organization.

WHO/CEGET (1987). *Atlas of the global distribution of schistosomiasis.* Bordeaux, Presses Universitaires de Bordeaux.

Yajima A et al. (2011). Moderate and high endemicity of schistosomiasis is a predictor of the endemicity of soil transmitted helminthiasis – systematic review. *Transactions of the Royal Society of Tropical Medicine and Hygiene*, 105:68–83.

IMPLEMENTATION

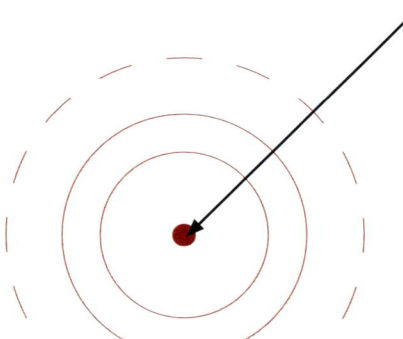

3.1 Community involvement

The participation of the community from the start of the planning phase is a key factor in the success of the control programme. Since improving children's health is the objective of the control activity, communities are normally supportive and ensure the necessary logistic support, provide additional practical information and help to underpin the long-term sustainability of the programme. Representatives of schools (teachers), community (parents, community leaders) and government should be informed as early as possible about:

- the epidemiological situation of schistosomes and STH in the area;
- the health risks posed by the infections;
- the likely benefits of the control programme.

Information should be provided to the community in a simple and clear style. Any percentages and prevalence must be presented in practical terms (for example, rather than saying that "there is 80% prevalence" it is preferable to say "in a class of 50 children, 40 are infected") and preferably in the local language(s). If the modalities of the intervention (for example, administration of drugs, provision of health education to

achieve behavioural change) and its short-term and long-term objectives (for example, improved health status, better performance in school) are fully explained at the outset, there will usually be strong family and community support for the programme.

A recent survey conducted in Viet Nam to assess the community perception of school deworming programmes showed complete satisfaction and a high level of support among students, teachers, health personnel and families. In addition, teachers were extremely willing to participate and to administer deworming drugs, even without remuneration (Mondadori et al., 2006).

3.2 Pilot phase – expansion phase

A phasing-in of control activities ensures that a large-scale programme runs smoothly and efficiently. All components of the programme should be tested in a pilot phase so that appropriate modifications can be introduced before the programme is expanded to a larger area. Testing is important; partners in the steering committee will benefit from the experience of working together and from working with

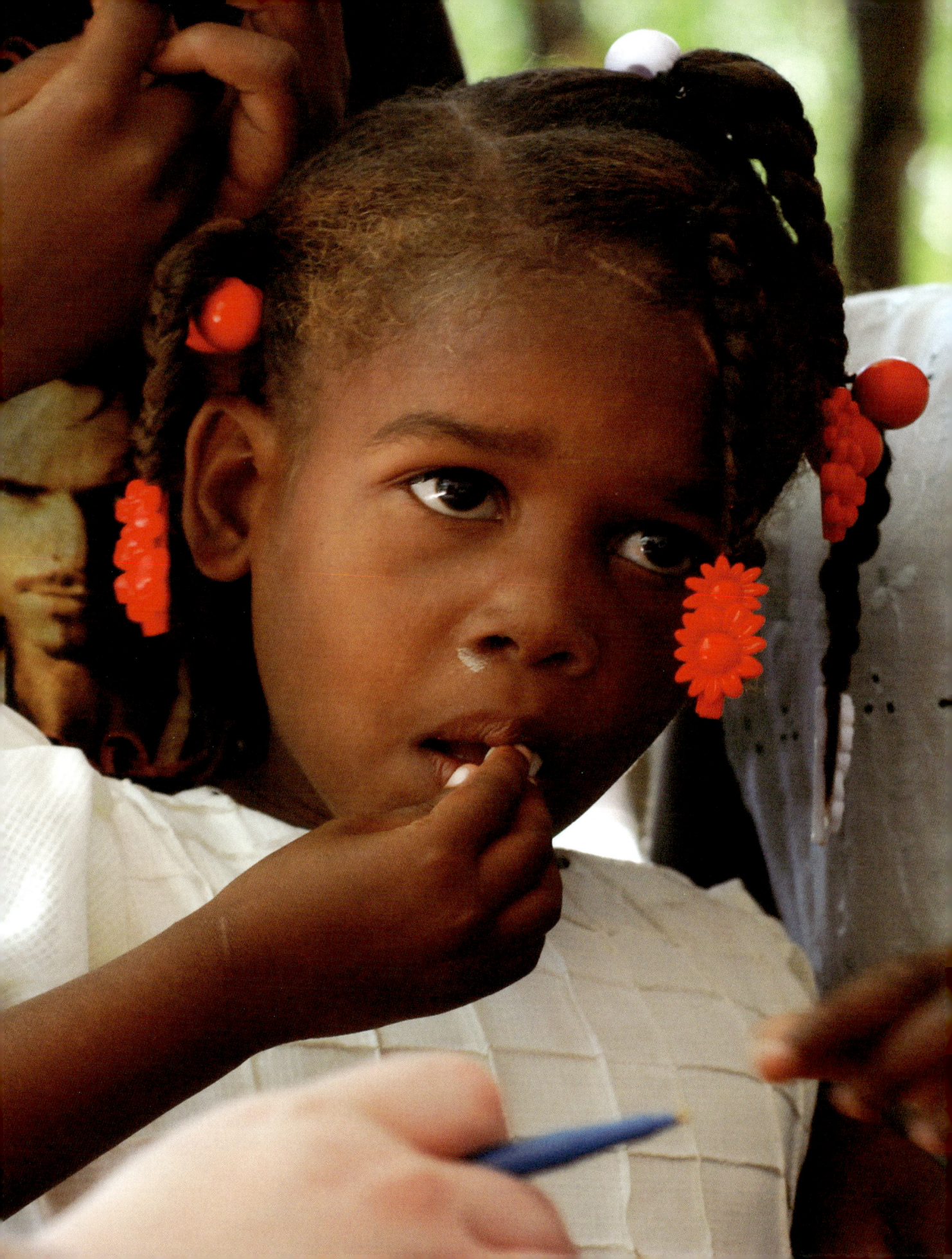

the different levels of the local health and school personnel participating in the control programme. Moreover, forms, questionnaires and educational material can be tested during the pilot phase, which will provide insight into the time and cost requirements of the different programme components. The accuracy of estimates (for example, of the number of non-enrolled children) can also be evaluated.

The pilot phase should, however, cover a sufficiently large population to provide useful insight into programme management. Ideally, at least 100 000 school-age children should be used in testing the procedures and the materials. Once the pilot phase has been completed and evaluated, the control programme can be scaled up to achieve countrywide coverage within 1–2 years.

3.3 Drug procurement, storage and distribution

The timely availability of drugs is essential for the effectiveness of the whole programme. Drug procurement is a key step in the implementation of control activities. For large programmes, drugs must be ordered well in advance because the quantities needed can make procurement a lengthy process – drug companies may not be able to provide large amounts of a drug in a short time.

3.3.1 Drug procurement

Whenever possible, drug procurement should be organized so that a quantity of tablets corresponding to one distribution round is always available as "buffer" stock. This will allow a drug distribution round to take place on a planned date despite possible delays in drug delivery or customs clearance. Drugs are best obtained in containers of 100 or 200 tablets; this reduces the need to open large containers and repackage the tablets in the smaller quantities needed for each school.

Local procurement
If good-quality anthelminthic drugs are locally produced, local procurement is the best option: it reduces transport costs, avoids the delays involved in importation and stimulates the local economy.

In most countries, the ministry of health has a specialized unit dealing with drug procurement. Whenever possible, this unit should be responsible for the procurement of drugs used in NTD control activities.

Example 1: Importance of community information in Malawi

Since 1999, Save the Children US, together with the Malawian Ministry of Education, has organized distribution of praziquantel in schools in Malawi.

In the first couple of years, children were suspicious of the treatment and less than half took the medication. Some children were scared because of the smell or large size of the tablets, or because their classmates felt dizzy after taking the pills. Community members were also suspicious, either because they did not trust medication in general or because they believed the pills were contraceptives. Furthermore, many community members considered schistosomiasis to be normal and did not understand the need for treatment. For these reasons, some parents forbade their children from attending school on treatment days.

To reduce scepticism and raise awareness of the importance of treatment, Save the Children sensitized the community through radio broadcasts that reminded parents of treatment dates and of the importance of treatment; community awareness meetings with senior chiefs, schools, surrounding villages and communities; notes to parents encouraging them to participate in the distribution; and notes to head teachers asking them to remind children of the importance and safety of the treatment.

To encourage children to take the medication on deworming days, Save the Children trained parents and other community members to participate and help teachers administer the treatment. Community members also performed plays, songs and poems to make treatment days more of a celebration and encourage the participation of all children.

The combined activities had a huge effect on coverage, which gradually increased to 82%. Communities are now familiar with the treatment and are convinced of its benefits. The participation of community members was a huge help to teachers who are often overwhelmed by the large classes that are a consequence of teacher shortages.

International procurement

If importation is the only option, purchasing and importing large quantities of drugs will be a complex undertaking involving many steps, governmental bodies and manufacturers. The document *Operational principles for good pharmaceutical procurement* (WHO/UNICEF/UNFPA/World Bank, 1999; see web link in *Annex 1*) presents a set of principles that can be adapted by individual governments and public or private organizations for developing procurement procedures.

Since 2011 GlaxoSmithKline and Johnson and Johnson have been donating respectively up to 400 million tablets of albendazole and 200 million tablets of mebendazole to control STH in school-age children.

Details on how to obtain donated deworming tablets are available at: http://www.who.int/intestinal_worms/en/index.html

Customs clearance of imported drugs is a critical step in the drug procurement process. The storage of drugs awaiting clearance is often expensive: contacting customs in advance of the date of arrival should help to speed up clearance and reduce costs. Early provision of the required import documentation (Certificate of analysis – Certificate of origin – pro-forma invoice/declaration of value, etc.) will also facilitate clearance. Where there are difficulties in procuring large amounts of drugs, programme managers may seek the assistance of WHO's Procurement Services (see Annex 1).

3.3.2 Drug quality

Drugs should be purchased from reliable pharmaceutical companies that are responsible for guaranteeing quality. National authorities should set up appropriate mechanisms, such as drug registration and/or prequalification of suppliers, in order to ensure that drugs procured for control campaigns are of the required quality. In addition, programme managers may need to confirm drug quality through independent analysis. National authorities should therefore have access to quality control laboratories for testing drug products.

The drug sample sent to the testing laboratory must contain at least 120 tablets. The tablets must be sent in the original sealed package: if the package contains 200 tablets, the entire package should be sent to the laboratory. Samples must be accompanied by a sample collection form (see *Annex 9*). The cost of quality testing can range from US$ 200 to US$ 1500 for each sample, depending on the testing site and the type of analysis required.

WHO has prequalified a number of quality control laboratories (see *Annex 1*) able to undertake testing at the request of countries that lack facilities. WHO can be contacted whenever programme managers suspect a drug quality problem.

3.3.3 Storage at central level

Drugs must be stored in a secure, cool and dry place. The ministry of health will probably have suitable facilities at central, regional and district levels. Space requirements for drug storage can easily be estimated. As an example, the space required to store 250 000 tablets, in containers of 200 tablets, is about 1 cubic metre. Drug transfer into and out of the central and peripheral storage facilities should be carefully recorded using the existing stock management system. If no satisfactory system is in place, programme managers should develop suitable forms and a recording system.

3.3.4 Distribution to regions, districts and schools

Before each round of drug administration takes place in the schools, an adequate quantity of drugs must be delivered to districts and schools. As far as possible, containers should be kept intact until received at the school. When the quantity of drugs to be sent to each district and school is calculated, the number should be rounded up to the next hundred to take into account unexpected requests and to avoid the need to open new containers at district level. Following these procedures is made easier if some of the drugs are procured in containers of 100 or 200 tablets.

Alternatively, at the district level, the original containers can be opened and the drugs divided into separate labelled containers to match the needs of each school. Counting tablets may seem to be a simple task, but it is easy to make mistakes. A small weighing scale can facilitate this task. Suitable containers and labels have to be provided by the programme since they are not usually available at district level.

Different countries have different drug distribution systems, so the specific modalities of distribution will need to be determined locally. The most important issues to consider are:

- making use, as much as possible, of the existing structures in the ministry of health;
- providing sufficient advance notice to storage and distribution facilities in the ministry of health for appropriate arrangements to be made.

Another efficient way of distributing drugs from the district level to schools is to combine the distribution with training activities (see *Example 2*). If at least one teacher from each school participates in training activities, the same teacher can carry the drugs back to the school.

3.3.5   Storage at peripheral level

The drug tablets will remain in the school for only a short period of time before being administered. The storage space (for example, cupboard in the school or in the local dispensary) should:

- be dry, to prevent moisture from affecting the appearance or efficacy of the drug;
- have secure doors to prevent theft;
- be protected against insects and other pests and from direct sunlight.

Drugs should not be stored in the same place as poisonous or toxic substances or chemicals such as kerosene and petrol.

3.3.6   Unused tablets

After treatment of the entire school-age population, some of the tablets may remain unused. This is not a problem because the public health goal is to achieve the highest coverage: having unused tablets is better than having children who were not treated because an insufficient number of tablets were provided to the school.

The number of unused tablets should be recorded and reported; this information will help managers to minimize overstocking in the following years. Because recovering unused tablets from each school tends to be more expensive than procuring new ones, the best use of the remaining drugs is to keep them for children who could not be present on the treatment day or to give them to the nearest health facility for treatment of individuals in other population groups (for example, preschool children or women of childbearing age).

3.4   Training

A "cascade" type of training ensures efficiency and standardization while allowing for local input (for example, to guide appropriate outreach activities). The first step is the organization of a central training team – a core of personnel to be responsible for organizing training activities at the regional level. Individuals trained at regional level will then train those at the district level. The number of training sessions needed in each district will depend on the number of schools and the distances involved. Sessions should be organized for a maximum of 40–50 teachers at a time from nearby schools.

The following sections summarize the major skills to be acquired by the various participants in the school deworming programme.

3.4.1   Programme managers

The experience of individuals who have already managed school-based helminth control programmes is invaluable. WHO is promoting exchange visits by managers from different countries and participation in international workshops to share their experience and different problem-solving approaches.

Example 2: Use of educational infrastructure to deworm schoolchildren in Lao PDR (Phommasack et al., 2008)

Lao's school-age children number approximately 1 014 000 (891 000 enrolled and 123 000 non-enrolled). The total number of registered primary schools is 2 600. These schools are grouped into clusters, each composed of 2–5 neighbouring schools.

In 2005, all cluster directors attended provincial training workshops on drug administration and health education. Each province conducted, on average, three 1-day workshops. The cluster directors then disseminated information to schoolteachers during regular weekly meetings.

Drugs and materials for the deworming campaign were delivered to each peripheral health unit by the Ministry of Health's network of trucks used for its regularly scheduled deliveries. After mebendazole arrived at the health units, each school cluster director collected it and delivered the appropriate number of tablets to each school for distribution. The teachers did not receive monetary compensation for administering the mebendazole tablets to the schoolchildren.

The coverage of school-age children in Lao PDR was estimated at 95.3% (99% for enrolled and 68.9% for non-enrolled). The cost for each treated child was US$ 0.12, most of which was accounted for by the training activities.

Since 2006, the Lao DPR school-based deworming campaigns have been repeated every 6 months at an estimated cost of US$ 0.04 per child. The reduction in cost was due to the fact that cluster directors did not need retraining after the first year.

For managers with limited experience of this type of helminth control programme, the best approach is "on-the-job" training. This is the rationale behind the suggestion that each programme start with a pilot phase. Managers can test different approaches in a pilot area in order to gain the necessary confidence to scale up to a regional or national level. WHO can be contacted by programme managers for technical support, guidelines, technical documentation and other materials (see *List of useful addresses provided in Annex 1*). When warranted, a visit by WHO personnel during specific phases of control activities can also be arranged.

3.4.2   Health personnel

The major skills to be acquired by health personnel during training are:

- communicating the rationale of the intervention to community leaders;
- distributing appropriate quantities of drug to each school;
- organizing drug administration in schools;
- supervising and supporting the teachers;
- dealing with adverse effects in children referred by teachers;
- reporting adverse effects.

Health personnel from the same areas as teachers should be invited to the training activities. Training sessions provide the opportunity to inform these individuals about the purpose and practical implementation of the school-based activities. Health personnel can support the activities of the teachers or, where their numbers are sufficient, undertake the drug administration themselves.

3.4.3   Teachers

The major skills to be acquired by teachers during training are:

- organizing drug administration in schools;
- using the weighing scale or the tablet pole to determine the number of praziquantel tablets to be administered;
- disseminating health education messages;
- reaching non-enrolled school-age children and providing them with deworming treatment;
- completing the forms for reporting (see model forms in *Annexes 7* and *8*);
- dealing with occasional mild side-effects and knowing which children to refer to health personnel;
- managing the drugs that remain after treatment.

Experience from several helminth control programmes has demonstrated the advantages of recruiting teachers for the implementation of programmes:

- Teachers are familiar with the children and know how to deal with them.
- Teachers are respected by the children and their families.
- Teachers are highly motivated and interested in health issues, particularly in improving the health status of children.

Anthelminthic administration is simple, especially when only mebendazole or albendazole is needed for a control programme. In some cases, large programmes have been organized without any formal training for the teachers (Montresor et al., 2007). When praziquantel is administered for the first time, however, it is strongly recommended that teachers be trained. One training session of a few hours is normally sufficient to train a group of 40–50 teachers. Each teacher should then be able to organize the drug administration in his or her school and to train other teacher colleagues in the school. Example 3 below shows the timetable and content of a training course conducted in Guinea in 2000. The programme targeted more than 2 million school-age children. During the course, each teacher was provided with the quantity of drugs and the health education material needed for his or her school. Training was organized in a large school to enable each participating teacher to practise drug administration in at least one class.

Trained teachers can administer deworming drugs and disseminate health education messages to the school-age population.

On average, it takes 20–30 minutes for a teacher to treat a class of 50 children. Treatment normally takes place during the school day, with the agreement of the ministry of education, and teachers in many countries therefore receive no financial remuneration for this task. Instead, 5–6 doses of the deworming drug are often provided to the teacher and her or his family as a non-monetary compensation. On the other hand, teachers attending training activities in the context of the school deworming programme would normally be reimbursed for the costs of travel and meals.

Example 3. Teacher/health personnel training session: school-based deworming programme in Guinea

Objective of the training activities – to enable teachers to organize an efficient drug administration, to deliver simple health education messages and to fill in the reporting forms correctly.

Trainers – education and health officers of the prefecture (geopolitical entity similar to the district)
Trainees – teachers and personnel of the peripheral health units
Place of training – primary school with at least 20 classes

Timetable

09:00–09:30	*Introduce aims of the school health programme*
09:30–09:45	*Discuss epidemiological results in the area*
09:45–10:00	*Discuss drug safety, process of referral, drug storage conditions*
10:00–10:30	*Questions and clarification*
10:30–11:00	*Coffee/tea break*
11:00–11:30	*Additional questions and clarification (including discussion of outreach activities)*
11:30–12:30	*Practical exercise – drug administration. Drugs administered to one demonstration class by the trainer and observed by the trainees. Teachers in groups of 3 or 4 administer drugs to the rest of the school.*
12:30–13:00	*Practical exercise – health education. Health education is provided to one demonstration class by the trainer and observed by the trainees. Teachers in groups of 3 or 4 provide health education to the rest of the school.*
13:00	*Distribution to each teacher of adequate quantities of drugs for his or her school.*

3.5 Delivering the intervention in schools

3.5.1 Treatment day

The administration of a single oral dose of albendazole (400 mg) or mebendazole (500 mg) is straightforward: each child receives one tablet. The teacher should ensure that each child swallows the tablet. Clean drinking-water should be available at the school on the treatment day.

If praziquantel is to be given in addition to one of the drugs mentioned above, each child must be given the correct number of tablets according to body weight (40–60 mg/kg

– see *Table 3.1*) or height (see *Figure 3.1*) and should stay in school for 2 hours after drug administration. If adverse effects occur during this time, the teacher should provide the simple measures suggested in *section 3.5.3*.

The tablets marketed as "chewable" are easily broken down and taste better. However, all formats of albendazole, mebendazole or praziquantel tablets can be broken down to facilitate administration to young children or to be chewed.

The names of the children who are absent on treatment day should be recorded by the teacher and these children should be treated when they return to school. Children who are

Table 3.1 Number of praziquantel tablets needed for different body weight ranges to provide a praziquantel dose of 40–60 mg/kg

Body weight range (kg)	No. of tablets of praziquantel (600 mg)
10–14.9	1
15–22.4	1½
22.5–29.9	2
30–37.4	2½
37.5–44.9	3
45–59.9	4
60 –75.0	5

ill on treatment days should not receive drugs. This is not because of any danger of adverse effects, but to prevent the potential misperception that the deworming medicine caused the illness. These children should be given the anthelminthic drug(s) later, when they are well again.

3.5.2 Use of the "tablet pole"

Height and weight are usually well correlated in children: a method for determining dosages of praziquantel that relies only on height (which can be readily measured) has been developed for use when weighing scales are not available.

The "tablet pole" is a long piece of wood marked with the height intervals corresponding to the number of tablets of praziquantel needed to treat school-age children for schistosomiasis. A child simply stands upright against the pole and the number of tablets corresponding to his or her height can be read from the pole. The tablet pole estimates the number of tablets for children who are between 94 cm and 190 cm tall.

The use of a tablet pole to determine dosage has several advantages over weighing children:

- it is cheaper than a weighing scale and has no moving parts that can break;
- it is simple and quick to use and requires no calculations;
- it is accurate and safe to use.

An analysis has shown that the doses of praziquantel given to 80–90% of children measured with a tablet pole are in the same range as doses that would have been determined by weighing. The remaining 10–20% of children receive a dose within an acceptable range for treatment of schistosomiasis (Montresor et al., 2001a; Montresor et al., 2005).

Figure 3.1 Use of the tablet pole

The pole has to be propped vertically against a wall, and each individual is classified, according to his or her height, in one of the seven intervals corresponding to the number of praziquantel tablets.

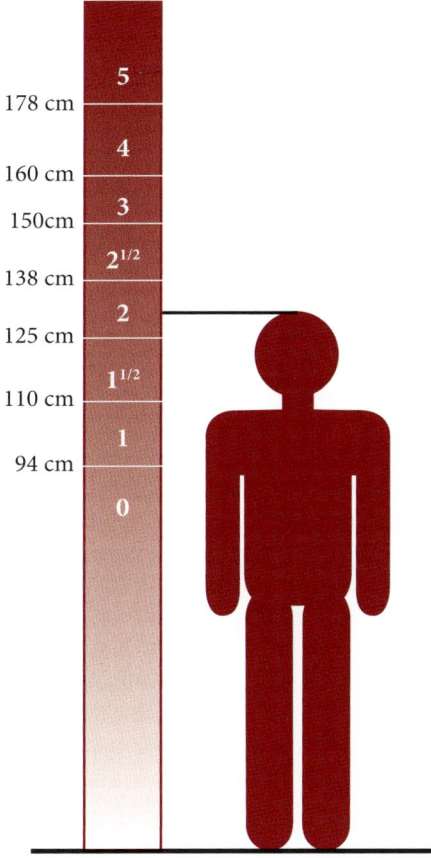

178 cm — 5
160 cm — 4
150 cm — 3
138 cm — 2 1/2
125 cm — 2
110 cm — 1 1/2
94 cm — 1
— 0

Implementation

The height thresholds of the pole are shown in *Figure 3.1*. A paper sample of the tablet pole is included with this book and can be used as a model for duplication. Many drug producers now include a paper sample of the tablet pole in their boxes of praziquantel.

3.5.3 Minimizing the impact of adverse events following anthelminthic treatment

An *adverse event* is any untoward medical occurrence that may present during treatment with a medicine but that does not necessarily have a causal relationship with this treatment. An *adverse drug reaction* is a response to a medicine which is noxious and unintended and which occurs at doses normally used in humans (WHO, 2002). These definitions indicate that there are events that are caused by the action of the medicine – the adverse drug reactions – as well as events that are not caused by the medicine and can simply be coincidental (that is, just temporally associated with the use of a medicine).

The deworming drugs used in school health programmes are effective, have an excellent safety record and are approved for use in school-age children. Cumulative experience of deworming millions of children worldwide shows that these drugs cause only rare, mild and transient adverse events or adverse drug reactions (Loukas & Hotez, 2006). Adverse drug reactions are generally reactions to degeneration of the worms that have been killed. Most of the side-effects observed in school programmes occur during the first rounds of implementation of the intervention; that is, at a time when children harbour more infections of high intensity. Mild abdominal pain, nausea, vomiting, diarrhoea and fatigue are the most frequently reported adverse effects and do not normally require medical treatment. However, it is important to address adverse events in advance by communicating clearly with community leaders: in some instances, rumours about the drug's lack of safety have resulted in a large number of children complaining of nonspecific symptoms and in a high number of referrals to the health units.

Briefly, the principal measures for minimizing the impact of adverse events and adverse drug reactions during anthelminthic treatment are the following (WHO 2011):

- Communicate clearly to the community leaders and parents the reasons for the school deworming intervention and information on the known adverse effects. Respond to questions and clarify doubts. Stress that:
    - adverse events will be minor and transient while preventive chemotherapy is highly beneficial;
    - an adverse event may occur at the same time as, or immediately after, the treatment, but this is not sufficient to attribute the cause to the drug administration;

- consumption of food before swallowing praziquantel tablets is not compulsory but is preferable because drug absorption is increased;
- Do not give the drugs to children who are ill on treatment day.
- Take immediate action in case of even minor adverse events: nausea, vomiting, diarrhoea and fatigue can be easily managed with inexpensive remedies (such as resting in a quiet room for a few hours, and providing water possibly mixed with sugar);
- In the first year of intervention, when infection intensities are highest, avoid triple therapy – the concomitant administration of albendazole, ivermectin and praziquantel – since adverse drug reactions are generally a reaction to the degeneration of the killed parasites. Administering the drugs on separate occasions avoids the simultaneous killing of large numbers of different parasites (schistosomes, STH and filariae) and thus reduces the probability of adverse reactions.

3.5.5 Health education/health promotion activities

The purpose of health education is to influence health-related behaviours by stimulating pupils' interest and guiding their efforts to improve their own health and that of their families and community. Health education should stress practical and basic information that will enable pupils to reduce the chances of exposure to infection. Close collaboration between education and health staff is necessary to identify behaviours that must be addressed in any particular community. Good standards of hygiene can be reinforced by having clean and functional latrines in the schools that are adapted to the needs of girls and boys.

The teachers are familiar with the concept of personal hygiene, so it is normally easy for them to transmit their knowledge to the children.

People must be helped to identify the specific behaviours that are likely to cause helminth infections so that such behaviours can be modified or avoided. Other information is also needed to encourage and enable pupils to adopt healthy practices. Information about values, beliefs and attitudes that may influence behaviours and conditions associated with helminth infections can be obtained from pupils and from parents by undertaking a knowledge, attitudes and practices (KAP) survey.

The availability of educational tools – documentation and other material – is important to help teachers promote health education among pupils. These tools should be designed to increase knowledge, build positive attitudes and values, dispel myths and encourage each child's capacity to practise healthy behaviours. Teachers can also be trained in health education/

health promotion activities that address personal hygiene, healthy nutrition, the dangers of smoking, the prevention of violence, and the prevention of HIV/AIDS and other sexually transmitted infections (and the discrimination related to these infections).

Common behaviours related to the transmission of helminth infections (WHO, 1996)

- Unhygienic habits that facilitate ingestion of parasite eggs or larvae:
  - not washing hands with clean water and soap before eating;
  - not washing raw vegetables and fruits with clean water before eating;
  - eating of soil.

- Behaviours that allow hookworms or schistosomes to penetrate the skin:
  - walking barefoot;
  - contact with contaminated fresh water.

- Behaviours that allow parasite eggs or larvae to contaminate the environment:
  - defecating anywhere other than a latrine;
  - urinating in fresh water.

- Behaviours that may result in continued transmission of infection:
  - failing to comply with treatment;
  - failing to improve sanitation facilities and management of faecal material.

Where endemic conditions warrant, other parasitic diseases not described in this book can easily be addressed during health education sessions and activities. For example, eating raw and undercooked fish, shellfish and meat can result in infection with flukes and tapeworms, and drinking untreated or unfiltered water can result in infection with guinea worm and bacterial and protozoan parasites.

Managers can see examples of health education/health promotion material on the WHO web site (see *Annex 1* for details).

In many countries, the teaching of these concepts is part of the normal school curriculum. This is convenient; the preventive measures are discussed during regular school hours and there is no need to develop, print and distribute additional material.

3.6 Integration with other activities

WHO recommends the integration of control activities for the different NTD diseases whenever possible (WHO, 2006), to help reduce costs and increase efficiency. The most productive form of integration is to use existing government structures and personnel to the greatest extent possible. Integration can be envisaged in several areas: drug administration, health education, training, data collection, and monitoring and evaluation.

In the area of *drug administration*, several forms of integration are possible that will produce further increases in efficiency, including:

- arranging the timing of drug administration for diseases treated with the same drug (such as STH infections and lymphatic filariasis) to comply with the recommended treatment interval for the different diseases;
- simultaneous provision of two drugs to the same group at risk for two different parasitic infections (for example, albendazole and praziquantel for schoolchildren);
- the use of existing infrastructure to reach specific risk groups (for example, vaccination campaigns to reach preschool-age children).

Integration is possible with other NTD control activities as well as with nutritional interventions (iron, iodine, vitamin A food supplements). This is particularly important: removing nutritional competition by the parasite means that nutritional supplements are better absorbed by the children (see *Table 3.2*).

In *health education*, the behavioural change messages provided to school-age children to reduce the transmission of helminth infections can be integrated with other similar hygiene messages (for example, improving oral hygiene to prevent caries and facial hygiene to prevent trachoma).

The *training sessions* conducted for teachers and health workers on deworming afford an opportunity to introduce additional messages to this group at very low cost.

In the area of *data collection*, costs could be reduced by forming teams to collect data for several purposes at the same time.

WHO provides technical support to endemic countries in the preparation of integrated Plans of Action for NTD control in which the intervention for the different diseases is implemented in an integrated way.

Table 3.2 Health interventions that can be integrated with a deworming programme targeted to school-age children.
Deworming strengthens the educational and nutritional benefits of nutritional interventions and can synergize disease control interventions.

	Possible accompanying activities	Indication	Intervention	Type of integration	References
Control of other NTDs	Active trachoma prevention	In areas where trachoma is endemic	Yearly administration of oral azithromycin (20 mg/kg)	The infrastructure used to distribute azithromycin can be used to distribute anthelminthics or vice versa.	Mathew et al., 2009
	Global Programme for the Elimination of Lymphatic Filariasis (GPELF)	In areas endemic for lymphatic filariasis (see also *section 2.5*)	Yearly administration of oral ivermectin (150 µg/kg) and albendazole (400 mg) or Yearly administration of oral diethylcarbamazine (6 mg/kg) and albendazole (400 mg)	Albendazole is included in prevention programmes for both STH and LF. The timing of the drug distributions is arranged in a way that best fits with the recommended interval of re-treatment for both diseases.	Ismail et al., 2001
Nutritional interventions	Iron and vitamin A supplementation	In areas where iron deficiency anaemia is a public health problem	Iron–folate tablets, 60 mg elemental iron and 0.40 mg folic acid (weekly)		Risonar et al., 2008
	Iodine supplementation	In areas of severe iodine deficiency and insufficient use of iodized salt	Oral iodized oil capsules 400 mg (every 1–2 years)	In schools, deworming can be administered at the same time as the nutritional and immunization interventions, by the same personnel, significantly reducing the costs	Peterson et al., 1999
	School nutrition programmes	In schools supported by the World Food Programme or by other food aid donors	Food supplementation (daily)		WFP/ UNESCO/ WHO, 1999
Immunization activities	School-based programmes	In countries where this activity is organized	Hepatitis B – DPT booster – human papillomavirus – Japanese encephalitis		School-based immunization (WHO web page *Annex 1*)

3.7 Outreach to non-enrolled school-age children

One of the most important challenges to school-based control programmes is the significant proportion of school-age children in many developing countries who do not attend school. These children have been shown to be more heavily infected than those who do go to school (Husein et al., 1996). Reaching non-enrolled school-age children is a challenge for any control programme. The extent of non-enrolment in each country can be obtained from reports by international organizations such as the United Nations Children's Fund

(UNICEF), the United Nations Educational, Scientific and Cultural Organization (UNESCO), and the United Nations Development Programme (UNDP). This information is also reported in the NTD country profiles edited by WHO (for web link see *Annex 1*).

The best means of reaching non-enrolled school-age children should be identified in each community on the basis of information supplied by local groups, women's organizations, religious leaders, community committees, family representatives and teachers.

Good results have been obtained by encouraging school-children to bring their non-enrolled siblings and friends to school on a "treatment day". Alternative methods are house-by-house administration of drug by volunteers, organization of special community gatherings or use of existing programmes targeting children (such as Child Health Days) to administer anthelminthics together with other health interventions (vaccinations, vitamin A, etc.). Announcement of treatment days by radio, television, music, theatre or "town criers" can convey the information to the population and help sustain coverage.

References

Husein MH et al. (1996). Who misses out with school-based health programmes? A study of schistosomiasis control in Egypt. *Transactions of the Royal Society of Tropical Medicine and Hygiene*, 90:362–365.

Ismail MM et al. (2001). Long-term efficacy of single-dose combinations of albendazole, ivermectin and diethylcarbamazine for the treatment of bancroftian filariasis. *Transactions of the Royal Society of Tropical Medicine and Hygiene*, 95:332–335.

Loukas A, Hotez P (2006). Chemotherapy of helminth infections. In: Brunton LL et al., eds. *Goodman and Gilman's The pharmacological basis of therapeutics*, 11th ed. New York, McGraw-Hill.

Mathew AA, Turner A, Taylor HR (2009). Strategies to control trachoma. *Drugs*, 69:953–970.

Mondadori E et al. (2006). Appreciation of school deworming program by parents in Ha Giang Province (Vietnam). *Southeast Asian Journal of Tropical Medicine and Public Health*, 37:1095–1098.

Montresor A et al. (2001a). Development and validation of a "tablet pole" for the administration of praziquantel in sub-Saharan Africa. *Transactions of the Royal Society of Tropical Medicine and Hygiene*, 95:542–544.

Montresor A et al. (2001b). Extending anthelminthic coverage to non-enrolled school-age children using a simple and low-cost method. *Tropical Medicine & International Health*, 6:535–537.

Montresor A et al. (2005). The WHO dose pole for the administration of praziquantel is also accurate in non-African populations. *Transactions of the Royal Society of Tropical Medicine and Hygiene*, 99:78–81.

Montresor A et al. (2007). Cost containment in a school deworming programme targeting over 2.7 million children in Vietnam. *Transactions of the Royal Society of Tropical Medicine and Hygiene*, 101:461–464.

Peterson S et al. (1999). Coverage and cost of iodized oil capsule distribution in Tanzania. *Health Policy and Planning*, 14:390–399.

Phommasack B et al. (2008) Coverage and costs of a school deworming programme in 2007 targeting all primary schools in Lao PDR. *Transactions of the Royal Society of Tropical Medicine and Hygiene*; 102:1201-1206.

Risonar MG et al. (2008). The effect of a school-based weekly iron supplementation delivery system among anemic schoolchildren in the Philippines. *European Journal of Clinical Nutrition*, 62:991–996.

WFP/UNESCO/WHO (1999). *School feeding handbook*. Rome, World Food Programme.

WHO (1996). *Strengthening interventions to reduce helminth infections as an entry point for the development of health-promoting schools*. Geneva, World Health Organization (WHO/SCHOOL/96.1).

WHO (2002). *The importance of pharmacovigilance*. Geneva, World Health Organization.

WHO (2006). *Preventive chemotherapy in human helminthiasis. Coordinated use of anthelminthic drugs in control interventions: a manual for health professionals and programme managers*. Geneva, World Health Organization.

WHO/UNICEF/UNFPA/World Bank (1999). *Operational principles for good pharmaceutical procurement*. Geneva, World Health Organization (WHO/EDM/PAR/99.5).

WHO (2011). *Assuring the safety of preventive chemotherapy interventions for the control of neglected tropical diseases*. Geneva, World Health Organization.

Example 4. Outreach to non-enrolled school-age children – the School Health Programme in Zanzibar (Montresor et al., 2001b)

The School Health Programme began in Zanzibar in 1994, under the leadership of the Ministry of Health. The programme covers 65 800 children. The estimated proportion of non-enrolled school-age children is 30%.

Objective of the outreach activities
To provide school-age children not enrolled in or not attending school with anthelminthic treatment and health education.

Strategy
During district-level teacher meetings, there was discussion on how to reach the 20 000 non-enrolled school-age children. Each group of teachers identified ways of informing families about the availability of anthelminthic treatment at the school on special "treatment days". A small sum of money (US$ 20) was given to each school to buy the necessary materials for outreach activities. Possible outreach approaches identified were:

(a) posters, handmade by pupils;

(b) traditional music group performing in the school on the treatment day;

(c) messages distributed via megaphones and radio, and by religious leaders, to inform the community about treatment days;

(d) child-to-child communication (enrolled children letting non-enrolled siblings and friends know about treatment days).

Results
The most cost-effective intervention was a combination of approaches (c) and (d). More than 60% of non-enrolled school-age children were treated at marginal additional cost.

MONITORING & EVALUATION

Photograph by WHO

4.1 Objective and cost of the monitoring and evaluation process

WHO sees monitoring and evaluation as an integral component of any control programme, essential to ensure both efficient implementation and maximal benefit for infected individuals, their families and communities (WHO, 2010). An appropriate evaluation system allows documentation of the programme's impact, informs current practice and guides future applications. It is important that the results of monitoring and evaluation activities be shared with communities, relevant government ministries and donors to maintain their interest in and support for the programme.

Monitoring and evaluation should be carried out with as little expense as possible, so as not to divert resources away from implementation activities. At the planning stage, it is recommended that approximately 5–10% of the programme budget be reserved for monitoring activities.

> WHO sees monitoring and evaluation as an integral component of any control programme, essential to ensure both efficient implementation and maximal benefit for infected individuals, their families and communities.

4.2 Suggested indicators

Monitoring and evaluation are based on the periodic collection and analysis of variables (indicators) with the aim of measuring changes occurring during programme implementation.

The suggested indicators for schistosomiasis and STH control programmes in school-age children can be grouped into three categories, as summarized in *Table 4.1*.

Process and performance indicators are used for monitoring, and performance and impact indicators for evaluation (see *Figure 4.1*).

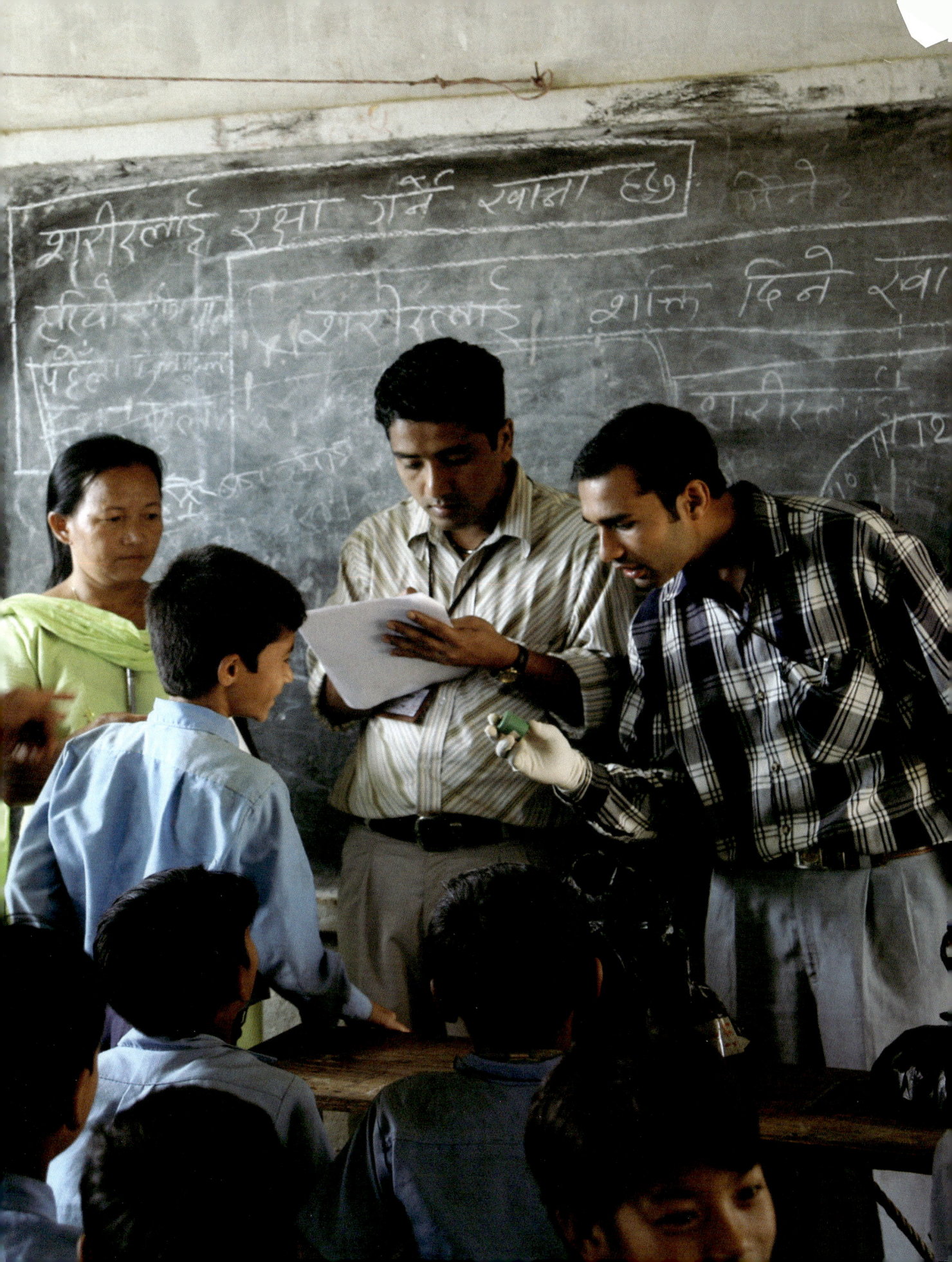

Table 4.1 Categories of indicators, their use and the frequency of their collection

Indicator category	Use	Frequency of collection
Process	Determine whether organizational elements of the control programme are in place and are functioning properly	At every drug administration round
Performance	Assess whether coverage of the control programme has reached its objective	At every drug administration round
Impact	Assess whether the health impact of the programme has been achieved	At baseline and every 2–3 years thereafter

Figure 4.1 Process, performance and impact indicators[a]

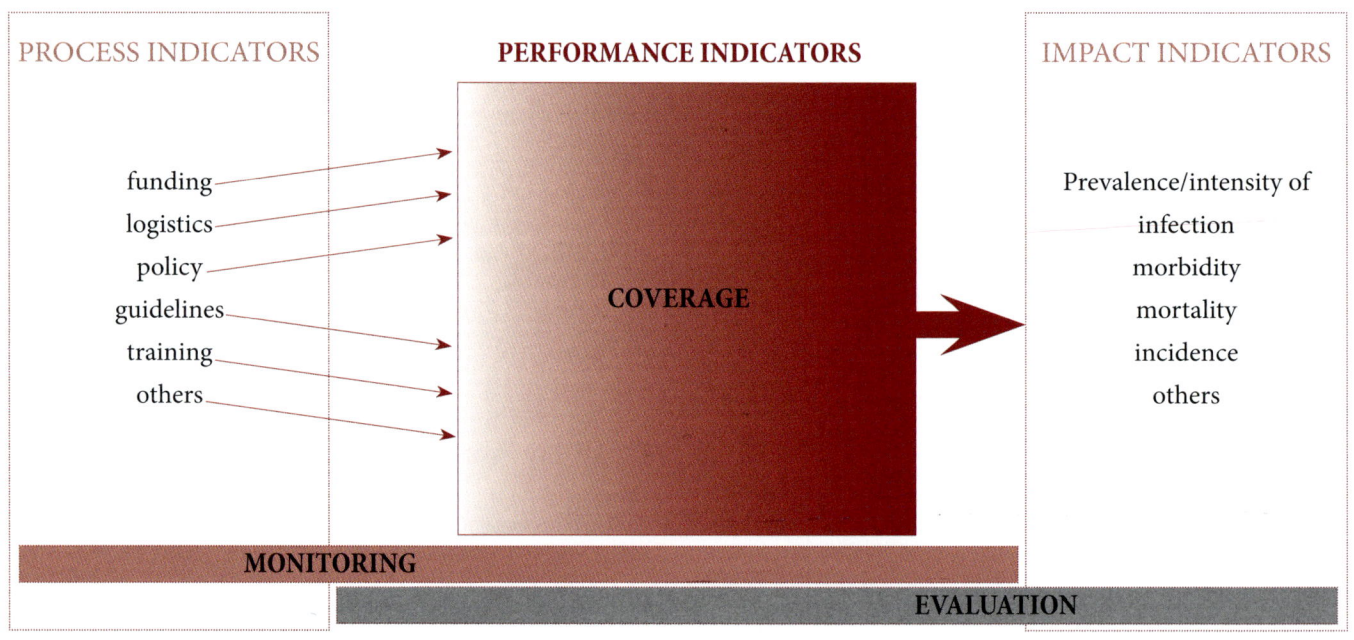

ᵃ Adapted from WHO, 2010.

Specific indicators in each category are listed in Tables 4.2, 4.3 and 4.4. Not all the indicators listed need to be collected – in fact, only a few are considered essential. Collection of additional indicators should be based on a clear rationale for their use and on resources available.

The data used to calculate indicators are normally collected using forms. Examples of suitable forms are given in *Annexes 4, 5, 6, 7, 8* and *9*; programme managers may decide to adapt these forms for their own particular programmes. Forms should be pretested before a control programme is initiated.

4.3   Process indicators

Once the control programme has started, the first monitoring activity involves assessment of the appropriateness of the drug procurement process, including timely arrival of drugs in the central pharmacy and peripheral storage depots, the appropriateness of the quantity and the expiry dates; the availability of weighing scales or tablet poles for the administration of praziquantel; the availability of reporting forms and education materials; the appropriateness and quality of the training and the attendance and the competences of the trainees. These data are normally derived from forms completed when the drugs and other materials are received in the central pharmacy and during training activities. Additional aspects may also be evaluated, such as the content of health education activities and drug storage conditions. The condition of latrines and the quality of water supplies in schools may also be monitored if their improvement is one of the objectives of the programme.

Time of collection of process indicators

Process indicators are normally more accurate if collected immediately after the relevant event (for example, for attendance at training sessions it is better to collect the list of participants immediately after the training). The process indicators, their calculation and use, and the expectations or goals of an effective deworming programme are summarized in *Table 4.2*.

Table 4.2 Process indicators, their calculation and use, and expectations or goals

Process indicator	Calculation	Use	Expectations or goals
Drug quality	Quality control report Expiry date of the drug received	To evaluate the efficiency of the drug procurement and storage process	Drug of appropriate quality received at least 2 years before the expiration date
Drug procurement	*Numerator*: Quantity of the drug received *Denominator*: Quantity of drug needed		100% of the needed drug is received in time
Drug distribution at peripheral units	*Numerator*: Number of (districts) schools receiving the drug supply in time and in appropriate quantity for the drug administration *Denominator*: Total number of (districts) schools targeted by the programme		Over 95% of the participating schools received the drug(s) at the appropriate time and in adequate quantity
Drug storage	*Numerator*: Number of tablets expired in the central storage facility *Denominator*: Number of tablets procured		Less than 5% of tablets are expired
Presence of tablet poles or weighing scales for praziquantel administration	*Numerator*: Number of (districts) schools receiving drug administration tools in time and in appropriate quantity for the campaign *Denominator*: Total number of (districts) schools covered by the programme	To evaluate the efficiency of the distribution of supporting materials	All schools receiving praziquantel also received tablet poles or weighing scales for distribution
Presence of reporting forms	*Numerator*: Number of (districts) schools receiving reporting forms in time and in appropriate quantity for the campaign *Denominator*: Total number of (districts) schools covered by the programme		All schools received reporting forms
Presence of health education materials	*Numerator*: Number of (districts) schools receiving health education materials in time and in appropriate quantity *Denominator*: Total number of (districts) schools covered by the programme		All schools received education materials in time to organize health education sessions
Presence of training materials	*Numerator*: Number of trainers receiving material in time and in appropriate quantity for organization of training sessions *Denominator*: Total number of (districts) schools covered by the programme		All trainers received training materials in timer to organize training sessions
Number of teacher training sessions	From programme forms	To determine whether sufficient training activities were given	At least one teacher in each school is trained with respect to implementing health education activities, administering the drug(s) and filling in the forms
Percentage of schools with at least one trained teacher	From programme forms		
Adequacy of the training	Teacher questionnaire, pre-test and post-test conducted during the training activities	To evaluate the need to revise training content	

Example 5: *Monitoring the process in Nepal* *(Bordignon & Deepak, 2003)*

Background and objectives

The World Food Programme (WFP) has been implementing a school feeding programme (SFP) in Nepal since 1996 with the objective of encouraging school enrolment as well as improving nutritional status of schoolchildren. The results of baseline parasitological surveys indicated a high prevalence and intensity of soil-transmitted helminth (STH) infections. Helminth control activities were therefore considered important in strengthening the benefits of the SFP in terms of the children's nutritional status and school performance. The following control measures were implemented in schools covered by the SFP:

- *twice-yearly anthelminthic administration to all schoolchildren;*
- *health education activities focusing on STH infections to all schoolchildren.*

Target

The deworming programme aimed to treat more than 75% of the school population (250 000 schoolchildren in approximately 2000 public primary schools in 12 districts).

Procurement of drugs

Albendazole (400 mg) was procured from a local manufacturer after evaluation of the drug quality and competitiveness of the price.

Training

In 1998, the Ministry of Health organized four training-of-trainers workshops for the district health and education staff from the 12 project districts. The participants, in turn, provided second-level training to schoolteachers and parents in each school in the programme.

Printing and distribution of posters

Some 3200 posters, illustrating how worms develop in the human body, how they can damage people's health, and how to prevent worm infection, and 3000 "flash cards" depicting sanitation scenarios, were printed for training and distributed to schools.

Administration of drugs

Albendazole tablets were transported to the primary schools through WFP channels, together with WFP foods. In each school, trained teachers administered albendazole tablets to schoolchildren.

Monitoring

Monitoring forms were developed to be filled in by teachers and district health officials for reporting data on training activities (e.g. number of teachers attending training), health education (e.g. number of education sessions conducted in each class) and drug administration (e.g. number of children receiving deworming).

Results

- *A quantity of drugs sufficient for all the schoolchildren targeted (plus 5% to cover incidentals) was received in Kathmandu WFP office in time for transportation to schools.*
- *100% of the schools had at least one trained teacher.*
- *More than 95% of the schools received sufficient drugs and health education materials.*
- *Over 90% of the enrolled schoolchildren received treatment.*

4.4 Performance indicators

Performance indicators assess the success of the programme in reaching the target population. The indicators evaluate the number and percentage of participating schools and the percentage of children receiving treatment and health education interventions. The data are normally obtained from the forms filled in during drug administration in the schools. The most important of these indicators is drug coverage (that is, the proportion of school-age children, both enrolled and non-enrolled, that received the drugs).

If data collected by forms are considered doubtful, a central team may conduct a "confirmation survey" in a small sample of schools, to compare the data reported by teachers with those directly collected in the schools (see *Example 6*).

Drug coverage is the key country-specific indicator collected by WHO to monitor progress towards the global target of treating 75% of school-age children in endemic countries (WHO, 2010). The data collected are summarized in the PCT databank (see *Annex 1*).

Time of collection of performance indicators

Performance indicators focus on the capacity of the programme to reach a large number of school-age children. To increase accuracy, these indicators should be collected immediately after the administration of a round of deworming drugs.

The performance indicators are listed in *Table 4.3*, which also specifies the numerators and denominators to be used in their calculation.

Table 4.3 Performance indicators, their calculation and use, and expectations or goals

Performance indicator	Calculation	Use	Expectations or goals
Percentage of schools participating in the programme	Numerator: Number of schools participating Denominator: Total number of schools in the in the targeted areas	Evaluating the extent of the programme and its relevance in the school system	>90% of the schools in the area participated
Number of tablets administered	From programme forms	To optimize the amount of drugs provided to the different schools	Over 90 % of the tablets are administred to children
Number of schools with a sufficient amount of drugs			Each school received enough drugs to treat all enrolled and non-enrolled school-age children
Number of tablets unused reported by teachers			No more than 10% of tablets are unused.
Coverage[a]	Numerator: Number of school-age children receiving the drug(s) Denominator: Total number of school-age children in the area of intervention	Determining the proportion of children receiving the intervention	>75% of school-age children have been treated
Percentage of classes participating in at least one health education activity	Numerator: Number of classes participating in at least one health education activity Denominator: Total number of classes in the area of intervention	Determining whether sufficient health education activities were undertaken	>90% of classes have participated in health education activities

[a] This indicator is the most important: reaching 75% of the school-age population has been identified by WHO as a minimal coverage target for endemic countries. Both numerator and denominator should include non-enrolled school-age children.

Example 6. Performance monitoring in Cambodia *(Sinuon et al., 2005)*

Background and targets

In 2002, Cambodia's Ministry of Health launched a deworming programme to deliver mebendazole (500 mg) and health education to at least 75% of its schoolchildren twice a year. The deworming programme was undertaken in two phases: the first phase targeted more than 1 million school-age children in 11 provinces and the second targeted the entire school-age population in the country (3.2 million children).

Method

The Ministry of Health monitored the programme coverage in two ways:

- *with standardized forms filled in by teachers in the 5850 schools in the country, and summarized at district and provincial level and transmitted to the Ministry of Health;*
- *with coverage-confirmation surveys conducted in 97 schools in 36 districts by the Ministry of Health central team; in each school visited, the team estimated the drug coverage – children who received drugs in each class were asked to stand up – and the data collected were then compared with the form filled in by the headmaster.*

Results

Forms – The Ministry of Health received more than 5800 forms from the schools, accounting for treatment of 2 774 564 schoolchildren (over 94% of enrolled children and 84% of the school-age population).

Confirmation survey – The coverage estimated by the confirmation survey differed from that in teachers' reports by an average of less than 5%. This validated the information from the teachers' forms and indicated that, in Cambodia, accurate assessments of coverage could be obtained from the teachers' reports alone.

4.5 Impact indicators

The main objective of a control programme is to reduce morbidity (by reducing the proportion of infected children, especially those with infection of moderate or heavy intensity). Impact indicators evaluate the effects of programme activities on improving health status. The indicators in this group are of two kinds:

- parasitological indicators directly related to drug action (e.g. reduction in prevalence and intensity of STH infections);
- indicators related to morbidity
  - caused by schistosomiasis (e.g. lesion of the urinary tract or liver);
  - caused by STH infection (e.g. malnutrition, anaemia) and its consequences (e.g. effects on school performance).

Impact indicators (including parasitological and morbidity indicators), their calculation and use, and related expectations or goals are summarized in *Table 4.4*.

4.5.1 Parasitological indicators

Regular collection of parasitological indicators provides a direct measurement of the effects of the control programme on the occurrence of helminth infections, and an indirect

measurement of the effectiveness of the programme in improving health status. In particular, these indicators show whether the proportion of infected children at baseline, and especially those with heavy-intensity infection, is declining.

Time of collection of parasitological indicators
At least 2 years of intervention are normally necessary before improvements in the health of school-age children can be measured with parasitological indicators.

Parasitological monitoring should be carried out just before a drug administration round (see *Figure 1.6*). Monitoring at this point will provide reliable information on reinfection occurring since the previous treatment, allowing the impact of previous treatment cycle(s) to be assessed. These data are normally collected in sentinel sites. A sample of schoolchildren should be selected in each of the ecological zones of the country. Details of the methodology for collecting parasitological indicators are given in *Chapter 5*. Treatment coverage data may help in the selection of appropriate areas for this assessment (that is, if only high-coverage areas are included in the sampling, the parasitological survey would probably overestimate the impact of the control programme and vice versa).

To facilitate the comparison of data from different countries, it would be useful to collect data in children of the same age; children in their third year of school are suggested (see also section 5.1). First-year children will not normally have been exposed to treatment, so this group would be more useful for evaluating whether transmission in the community has been reduced. Unless ther are deworming interventions targeted to pre-school aged children.

4.5.2 Morbidity indicators

Improvements in morbidity indicators are likely to be seen only where a control programme has been in effect for some time. A list of the possible signs of morbidity in schistosomiasis and STH infections is given in *Table 1.3*. The collection of morbidity indicators requires experienced personnel and accurate instruments (for example, ultrasound equipment, stadiometer, digital haemoglobinometer). Collection is therefore expensive and difficult. If programme resources do not permit the purchase of such specialized equipment for use by trained personnel, it is wiser *not to*

measure such indicators than to measure them without the necessary precision.

As an alternative, programme managers could establish collaboration with specialized research institutions that can collect accurate morbidity data at no cost to the programme and then use the data for research purposes. It is suggested that funds intended for control activities should not be used for research purposes.

Details on the methods for assessing morbidity due to schistosomiasis may be found in *Ultrasound in schistosomiasis* (Richter et al., 2000). Methods for nutritional measurements (haemoglobin, height and weight) can be found in *Measuring change in nutritional status* (WHO, 1983).

Measurement of morbidity indicators can be carried out at the same time as parasitological monitoring (see child form in *Annex 5*) or at other times.

Example 7. Parasitological monitoring in the Seychelles *(Shamlaye, 2003)*

Background
A strategy to reduce morbidity and, in the long term, transmission of intestinal parasites, was implemented in the Seychelles in 1993. Drug distribution activities through health facilities targeted 20 000 children. The strategy focused on deworming primary and secondary school-age children three times a year, on health education, and on improvements in sanitation and water supply.

Targets
The programme aimed to reduce soil-transmitted helminth (STH) infections to a level at which morbidity would no longer be a public health problem (<1% prevalence of heavy-intensity infections).

Method
Coverage data were collected after each round of deworming. In addition, a parasitological survey was conducted every 2 years on a sample of 1000 children; the stool specimens were examined using the Kato-Katz technique.

Results
Programme coverage was estimated at 99.4%; parasitological monitoring yielded the results shown in the table below.

STH	1993		1994		1996		1998	
	Prevalence	% heavy infection	Prevalence	% heavy infection	Prevalence	% heavy infection	Prevalence	% heavy infection
A. lumbricoides	17.7	1.0	4.4	0.1	3.7	0.1	0.9	–
T. trichiura	53.3	1.1	27.3	0.7	21.5	0.1	5.3	–
Hookworms	6.3	0.6	4.2	0.1	1.6	0.1	1.1	–
Prevalence of any STH infection	60.5	2.7	33.8	0.9	24	0.3	7.3	–

After 5 years of intervention, the number of infected children was reduced by more than 87% and, more importantly, no more heavily infected children were found. This was probably a consequence of the concomitant and rapid socioeconomic development of the country, legislation to enforce implementation of sanitation throughout the country, and the high level of school attendance which significantly facilitated the programme.

Table 4.4 Impact indicators, their calculation and use, and expectations or goals

Impact indicators	Calculation[a]	Use	Expectations or goals
(a) Parasitological indicators			
Overall prevalence of any STH infection	*Numerator*: Number of children positive for any of the three STH infections	To measure the effectiveness of the control measures	Reduction of prevalence over time, especially where drug interventions are combined with behavioural and environmental improvements
Prevalence of each STH (*A. lumbricoides*, *T. trichiura* and hookworm)	*Numerator*: Number of children with each STH infection	To assess the need to change the frequency of treatment (for details, see *section 4.7*)	
Prevalence of intestinal schistosome infections	*Numerator*: Number of children with intestinal schistosome infection		
Prevalence of any haematuria or parasite eggs in urine	*Numerator*: Number of children with any haematuria or parasite eggs in urine		
Overall proportion of "heavy-intensity" infection with any STH	*Numerator*: Number of children heavily infected with any of the three STH[b]	To measure the effectiveness of the control measures in reducing heavy-intensity infections	
Proportion of "heavy-intensity" infections with each STH	*Numerator*: Number of children heavily infected with each STH[b]		The proportion of children heavily infected has been reduced to less than 1% in 2–3 years
Proportion of "heavy-intensity" intestinal schistosome infections	*Numerator*: Number of children heavily infected with intestinal schistosomes[b]	To assess the need to change the frequency of treatment (for details, see *section 4.7*)	
Proportion of visible haematuria or "heavy-intensity" urinary infection	*Numerator*: Number of children with visible haematuria or heavily infected with urinary schistosomes[b]		
(b) Morbidity indicators			
Proportion of children with clinical signs or symptoms (e.g. lesion of urinary tract or in the liver)	*Numerator*: Number of children with a specified clinical sign or symptom *Denominator*: total number of children examined for that clinical sign or symptom	To determine the effects of the programme on health status	The proportion of children with morbidity resulting from STH infection and/or schistosomiasis has been reduced to less than 1% in 5 years.
Percentage of children with anaemia[c]	*Numerator*: Number of anaemic children (Hb <115 g/litre) *Denominator*: Total number of children investigated for haemoglobin status		
Percentage of children with severe anaemia[c]	*Numerator*: Number of children with Hb <70 g/litre *Denominator*: Total number of children investigated for haemoglobin status		

[a] For all parasitological indicators, the denominator is the number of children from whom the parasitological data have been collected.

[b] Classes of intensity are presented in *Table 5.2*.

[c] Confirm Hb thresholds for specific child populations participating in the deworming programme (e.g. at different altitudes) (WHO, 2001).

4.6 Additional indicators

In certain circumstances, the collection of additional indicators may be warranted. The following four indicators serve as examples only; others can be formulated to reflect special needs or concerns.

Knowledge–Attitudes–Practice
An assessment of changes in knowledge, attitudes and practice (KAP) as a result of the health education activities can be valuable for the development of further health education messages. This evaluation can be done either with questionnaires or by observing behaviours (for example, hand-washing with soap). Assessment is difficult and programme managers can ask the support of an educational expert.

Assessment of drug efficacy
Anthelminthics are extremely effective in the treatment of worm infections but do not normally kill 100% of the worms (Keiser & Utzinger, 2008). Anthelminthic efficacy can be evaluated by calculating the *egg reduction rate* (reduction in the mean epg after treatment). When evaluating drug efficacy, data for calculating this indicator should be collected no later than 3 weeks after drug administration to avoid counting any possible cases of reinfection that might have occurred. Thus far, no instances of reduced efficacy of albendazole, mebendazole or praziquantel have been confirmed in humans. However, WHO/NTD (see *List of useful addresses in Annex 1*) should be consulted if programme managers suspect a reduction in drug efficacy: drug resistance may have developed, but expert investigation is essential. The topic is dealt with in *Report of the WHO informal consultation on monitoring of drug efficacy in the control of schistosomiasis and intestinal helminths* (WHO, 1999); a working group on the issue has been established by WHO and a standard protocol for evaluating drug efficacy has been developed (for additional details, WHO/NTD can be contacted at the address given in *Annex 1*).

Safe water supply and adequate sanitation
Where construction, repair and maintenance of a water supply or latrines have been a component of the control programme or are conducted in the area covered by the programme by other groups, it may be appropriate to include a specific assessment of their presence, adequacy and conditions. The additional process indicators should be formulated to reflect the specific nature of the sanitation interventions (for example, "schools with a sufficient number of functioning toilets" if this was the aim of the intervention). In general, obtaining data on safe water and sanitation coverage within the community and within the school would be helpful to understand the environmental factors affecting any change in the prevalence.

School effects
Indicators under this heading include school attendance, absenteeism, retention and school achievement. The success of school-based activities in achieving outreach to other risk groups, or even to the community as a whole, can also be ascertained.

4.7 When to reduce the frequency of drug administration

After a number of deworming rounds with good coverage, parasitological indicators collected at sentinel sites will show a reduction in the prevalence and intensity of infection in the target population. It is not possible to predict whether this reduction will be permanent or whether infection will return to original levels soon after the interruption of regular treatment.

The table in *Annex 10* is intended to help managers of control programmes decide whether and how to reduce the frequency of deworming interventions. Since very few programmes have documented the details on reducing the frequency of drug administration, the table will be updated as additional data become available.

The suggested measures apply if the coverage of the intervention has been constantly over 75%. If satisfactory coverage has not been reached, it is suggested to defer the decision to reduce the frequency of intervention until this condition has been satisfied.

These thresholds are more restrictive than those presented in *Tables 2.2* and *2.3* because prevalence is collected in a situation in which anthelminthic drugs have been administered for over several years. In this situation, even a moderate prevalence (of, for example, 20%) indicates that the parasites maintain transmission capacity despite intense drug pressure, and this is predictive of a rapid return to high levels of prevalence if the drug intervention is interrupted. (The situation is similar to that described in *section 2.5* of a school programme starting in an area where there has been distribution of albendazole for the elimination of lymphatic filariasis for 5-6 years).

Sentinel site monitoring activities should continue annually after the reduction in the frequency of drug administration.

If sentinel site monitoring shows that the prevalence remains low for 4 years despite the reduction in frequency of drug administration, a further reduction could be applied.

If monitoring indicates that prevalence tends to return to the original levels (recrudescence of the infections), reintroduction of the original treatment schedules will be warranted.

Example 8. Control of schistosomiasis in Cambodia (Sinuon et al., 2007)

Background and targets

In Cambodia, schistosomiasis is known to be transmitted in two provinces with approximately 80 000 individuals at risk of infection. In 1994, the baseline prevalence of infection was estimated to be between 73% and 88%. In addition, cases of severe morbidity (for example, hepatosplenomegaly, delayed puberty) and mortality due to Schistosoma mekongi infection were common in the area. In 1994, the Ministry of Health began a schistosomiasis control programme, delivering annual chemotherapy with praziquantel to the entire population of the endemic area. This simple control measure, applied over a period of 10 years, resulted in a dramatic reduction in the prevalence of the disease as illustrated in the graph below. Cases of severe morbidity due to schistosomiasis were no longer observed and only three cases of infection of light intensity were reported in 2005.

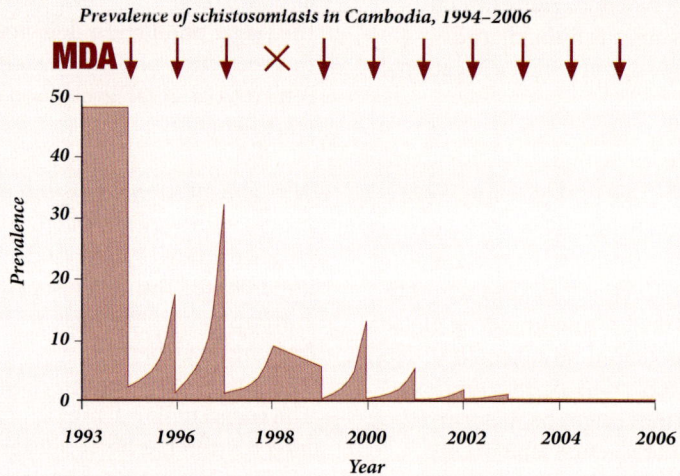

Prevalence of schistosomiasis in Cambodia, 1994–2006

In order to keep the disease under control and to reduce the cost of the yearly mass distribution, the Cambodian Ministry of Health decided to reduce the frequency of mass drug administrations (to every 2 years) and to monitor the possible recrudescence of infection by periodic serological screening using a very sensitive ELISA test (Ohmae et al., 2004).

References

Bordignon GP, Deepak RS (2003). Deworming Programme in Nepal supported by the World Food Programme. In: eds. Crompton DWT et al. *Controlling disease due to helminth infections*. Geneva, World Health Organization: 87–92.

Keiser J, Utzinger J (2008). Efficacy of current drugs against soil-transmitted helminth infections: systematic review and meta-analysis. *Journal of the American Medical Association*, 299:1937–1948.

Ohmae H et al. (2004). Schistosomiasis mekongi: from discovery to control. *Parasitology International*, 53:135–142.

Richter J et al (2000). *Ultrasound in schistosomiasis: a practical guide to the standardized use of ultrasonography for the assessment of schistosomiasis-related morbidity*, World Health Organization, Geneva.

Shamlaye N (2003). The Seychelles experience in controlling helminth infections. In: Crompton DWT et al., eds. *Controlling disease due to helminth infections*. Geneva, World Health Organization:239–248.

Sinuon M et al. (2005). Financial costs of deworming children in all primary schools in Cambodia. *Transactions of the Royal Society of Tropical Medicine and Hygiene*, 99:664–668.

Sinuon M et al. (2007). Control of *Schistosoma mekongi* in Cambodia: results of eight years of control activities in the two endemic provinces. *Transactions of the Royal Society of Tropical Medicine and Hygiene*, 101:34–39.

WHO (1983). *Measuring change in nutritional status*. Geneva, World Health Organization.

WHO (1999). *Report of the WHO informal consultation on monitoring of drug efficacy in the control of schistosomiasis and intestinal helminths*. Geneva, World Health Organization.

WHO (2001). *Iron deficiency anaemia: assessment, prevention and control: a guide for programme managers*. Geneva, World Health Organization.

WHO (2010). *Monitoring drug coverage for preventive chemotherapy*. Geneva, World Health Organization.

Collection of
EPIDEMIOLOGICAL DATA
in
SENTINEL SITES

Photograph by WHO

From the start of any control programme, a system must be established for the periodic collection of parasitological data for monitoring purposes. One of the most efficient methods of collecting epidemiological data is to use sentinel sites.

5.1 Concept[1]

From the start of any control programme, a system must be established for the periodic collection of parasitological data for monitoring purposes. One of the most efficient methods of collecting epidemiological data is to use sentinel sites. In a school-based control programme, a sentinel site is a school in which stool and urine specimens from approximately 50 children in the third-year class are investigated.

The sentinel site method assumes that changes in the prevalence and intensity of schistosomiasis and STH infections in a limited number of sentinel sites (schools) will provide sufficient information on the programme's progress in the entire area.

5.1.1 Location of sentinel sites

To ensure that the control programme is adequately monitored, sentinel sites should be located in each homogeneous ecological zone (see *section 2.1*). Each such zone normally covers several districts in a country (see *Example 9*) and can also be composed of non-contiguous districts.

5.1.2 Number of sentinel sites

The number of sentinel sites is normally proportional to the number of school-age children living in each zone. One sentinel site for every 200 000–300 000 targeted children is suggested; the proportion can be increased in the case of small-scale interventions.

The suggested ratio of sentinel sites to target population takes into consideration the fact that cluster sampling is used (50 children examined in each school) in several control programmes (Belizario et al., 2009; Koukounari et al., 2007) and offers several advantages:

---

[1] WHO can be contacted to obtain technical support about the organization of sentinel site surveys (see List of useful addresses in *Annex 1*).

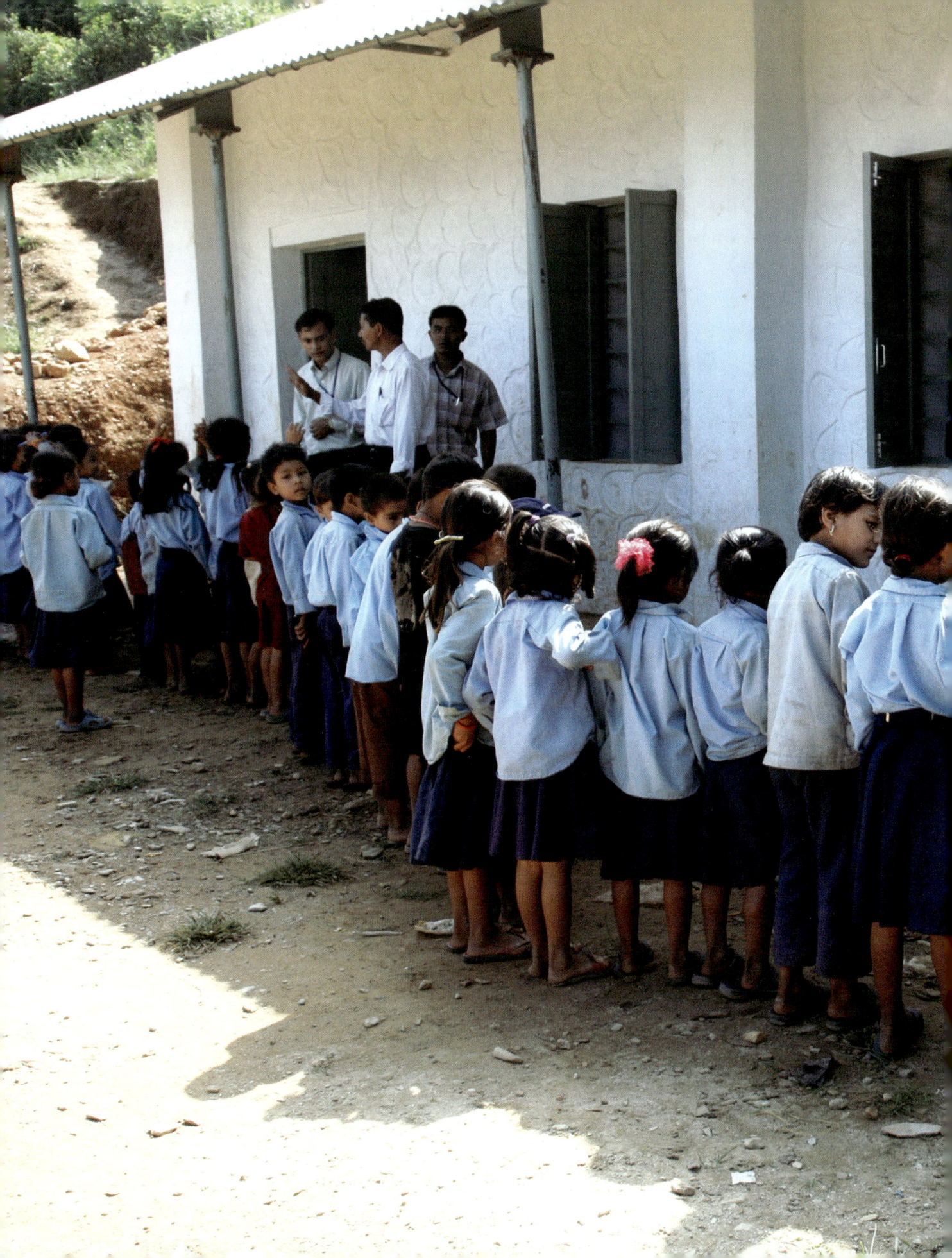

- It allows estimates to be obtained with:
  - an absolute precision of 5%;
  - a confidence level of 95%.

  which is sufficient for monitoring purposes (Lwanga & Lemeshow, 1991).

- It keeps the cost of the monitoring process under 10% of the total budget.
- It represents all the ecological zones.

5.1.3 Method for the selection of sentinel sites

A stratified sampling method should be used to select the schools that will serve as sentinels. For example, if 5 sentinel schools are needed in an ecological zone with a total of 20 districts, a number should be assigned to each district and a table of random numbers used to select 5 districts. Alternatively, a lottery method can be used: the names of all 20 districts are written on separate pieces of paper which are placed in a container – 5 names are then drawn from the container.

Once the 5 districts are selected, one school in each district can be randomly selected by the local team (using the list of schools that is normally available at district level). *Care should be taken to include all schools in the district, including private, religious and other special schools, in the sampling frame.*

In principle, the same sentinel schools should be used to monitor the impact of the programme over the years. In some cases, however, repeating the data collection in the same schools has resulted in increasing awareness in those schools and therefore in a reduction in transmission that does not reflect the situation in the other (unsampled) schools. To avoid this bias, 50% of the sentinel schools can remain the same over the years while the location of the remaining 50% is changed every year.

Once the number and location of the sentinel sites have been selected, health and education authorities – at regional, district and village levels – and the relevant community authorities should be contacted for permission to visit the schools and collect the stool and/or urine specimens. There should be meetings with those involved to explain the purpose of the deworming programme and of the survey, and the expected benefits for the children and the community.

5.1.4 Informing schools

A letter of introduction should be sent well in advance to the selected schools to explain the details of the survey and inform the principals of the date of data collection. The survey team leader (possibly accompanied by a member of the district staff of the ministry of education) should make an appointment to arrive at the school in the morning. He or she should introduce the team to the school staff and explain the aim of the exercise. *Parents must have been informed that they can withdraw their children from the survey at any time and without disadvantage for either the children or themselves.* After the data analysis, meetings should be held to inform all those involved about the preliminary results of the survey.

5.1.5 Selection of children

In each sentinel school, a lottery method should be used to select 50 children from among those in third-year classes. If the number of children in the third year is less than 50, another class of an older age group should be selected to give a total of at least 50 children.

5.2 Personnel needed

The following sections describe the skills needed by the field team who will collect stool and/or urine specimens, perform the laboratory investigation and compile the results.

A field team should be composed of at least a team leader, two or three laboratory technicians and one auxiliary worker.

The team leader is normally from the central level to ensure uniformity in the collection of data. Laboratory technicians could be from the central level or preferably from the regional (or provincial) hospital, and the auxiliary worker is normally locally recruited from a health unit near to the school.

Assistance from a local (district) education officer is useful in helping to locate the selected schools and in introducing the health team to the school personnel. This officer can also assist in data recording and in managing the flow of children through the various data-collecting stations, possibly with the help of the teachers in each school.

This team should be able to collect and analyse specimens from at least 50 children in a sentinel site in one or two days.

Tasks and responsibilities of team members
The team leader is responsible for:

- contacting community leaders and local health and school personnel to obtain permission to collect and analyse data from the schoolchildren;
- organizing the logistics for the collection of stool and urine specimens;
- periodically checking the completion of the data forms;

Example 9. Sentinel site monitoring in Burkina Faso *(Touré et al., 2008)*

General information on the control programme

Objective – 80% reduction of the prevalence of schistosome in the first two years of activity.

Intervention – Treatment with praziquantel and albendazole every other year.

Target – School-age population (5–15 years old)[1] in the entire country (approximately 3.6 million children).

Ecological zones – Burkina Faso can be divided into three main ecological zones:

- Sahelian in the north (approximate target population 300 000);
- Sahelo-Sudanese in the centre (approximate target population 2.6 million);
- Sudanese in the South East (approximate target population 700 000).

Selection and location of sentinel sites

Based on the distribution of the resident population in the different ecological zones:

- 6 schools were selected as sentinels in the Sahelian area;[2]
- 8 schools were selected in the Sahelo-Sudanese area;
- 3 schools were selected in the Sudanese area.

The location of the sentinel schools is shown in the figure below.

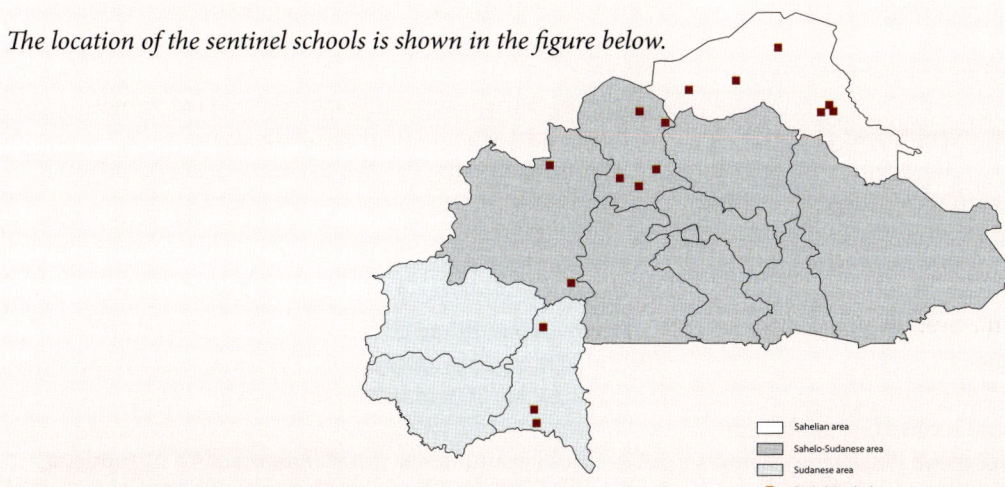

Results of the monitoring process

The table below shows the epidemiological changes in the prevalence of Schistosoma haematobium measured in the first 2 years of the intervention.

Prevalence of schistosomiasis collected in sentinel site in Burkina Faso at baseline (2004) and 2 years after first treatment

	Prevalence(%)	
	Baseline (2004)	2 years after treatment (2006)
Sahelian area	89.4	11.6
Sahelo-Sudanese area	51.1	12.3
Sudanese area	34.3	1.5
National prevalence	59.6	7.7
Proportion of infections of high intensity	25.2	2.0

*Two years after the first treatment, the intervention had resulted in an **87%** reduction in prevalence and a **92%** reduction in the number of high-intensity infections compared with baseline.*

---

[1] The standard definition of school age (5–14 years) was extended to cover the entire schooling age in Burkina Faso (5–15 years).

[2] The Sahelian area was over-sampled in comparison with the number suggested in paragraph 5.1.2 because it was considered to be the most endemic zone and the local managers wanted to obtain more detailed information from this zone.

- periodically checking the quality of the work performed by the laboratory technicians;
- summarizing the data and preparing preliminary reports for health authorities and the communities involved;
- delivering treatment in the schools being investigated.[1]

The laboratory technicians are responsible for:

- collecting the stool and urine specimens in labelled containers;
- preparing and examining stool and urine specimens according to standard procedures;
- recording results.

The auxiliary worker is responsible for:

- ensuring a clean working environment;
- ensuring the continued availability of clean containers, clean slides and other material for the Kato–Katz and filtration techniques (see also *paragraphs 5.4.1* and *5.4.2*);
- measuring and recording children's height and weight (optional);
- ensuring the safe disposal of contaminated material.

The assistance of one or two teachers in recording each child's name, age and sex and in managing the flow of children through the data-collecting stations is highly desirable.

5.3 Collection of biological specimens

Each child in the selected class should receive one container for a stool specimen (and another for urine if *S. haematobium* infection is to be investigated).

When stool containers are distributed, the amount of stool needed should be indicated with a demonstration of how to put it into the container using a wooden stick. The containers should be distributed to the schoolchildren either on the day of collection or during the previous day. Generally , the number of specimens returned is independent of the timing of container distribution, but the first option simplifies the work by requiring only one visit to each school. The cultural appropriateness of this approach must be checked before the start of the survey. Urine containers should be distributed on the day of the survey.

Additional data collected from the school (on the number of pupils enrolled and water and sanitation conditions) can help with the interpretation of the epidemiological data (see *Annex 4*).

The simplest way to collect data (personal and nutritional) and specimens (urine and stool) is to organize a flow of children through "stations" where specific data are collected (see *Figure 5.1*). Every child should be provided with a form (see *Annex 5* for an example) to carry through the stations where personal data are registered, urine is filtered or tested with reagent strips, and stool containers are collected and labelled.

An ID number must be allocated to each child and used to mark his or her sample containers and form. This practice also allows identification of the child in the event that any special treatment or care is needed.

Microscopic examination of stool specimens can be performed at the school or the stool samples can be transported to a local laboratory for examination.

No fixative (such as formalin) should be added to the specimen: fixatives may damage hookworm eggs and dilute the specimens, hampering the calculation of infection intensity.

5.4 Laboratory examinations

Parasitological diagnosis of schistosomiasis and STH infections is made by examining urine and/or stool specimens for the presence of helminth eggs.

5.4.1   Stool examination (for *A. lumbricoides*, *T. trichiura*, hookworms, *S .mansoni* and *S. japonicum*)

The Kato–Katz technique (WHO, 1991; WHO, 1994) involves the microscopic examination of a known amount of faecal material. Egg counts give an indirect measure of the worm burden: the higher the egg count, the greater the number of worms infecting the individual concerned. Ideally, the specimens should be collected in the morning and processed and examined in the afternoon of the same day. This simplifies the daily routine and reduces the number of containers and slides needed since they can be cleaned and reused. Microscopic examination is best performed within 1 hour of the preparation of slides: hookworm eggs, in contact with the glycerol in the cellophane strip, tend to become transparent over time and may be overlooked.[2]

---

[1] Following the principle of "no survey without service", the survey team should be equipped with drugs to treat schistosomiasis and STH infections. Children found to be suffering from other diseases should be referred to the nearest health centre.

[2] A description of the materials and reagents needed, and of the procedure, is given in *Bench aids for the diagnosis of intestinal parasites* (WHO, 1994), which is also available online (see plate 3, slides 48–55).

Figure 5.1 Flow of the children through the different stations during the data collections

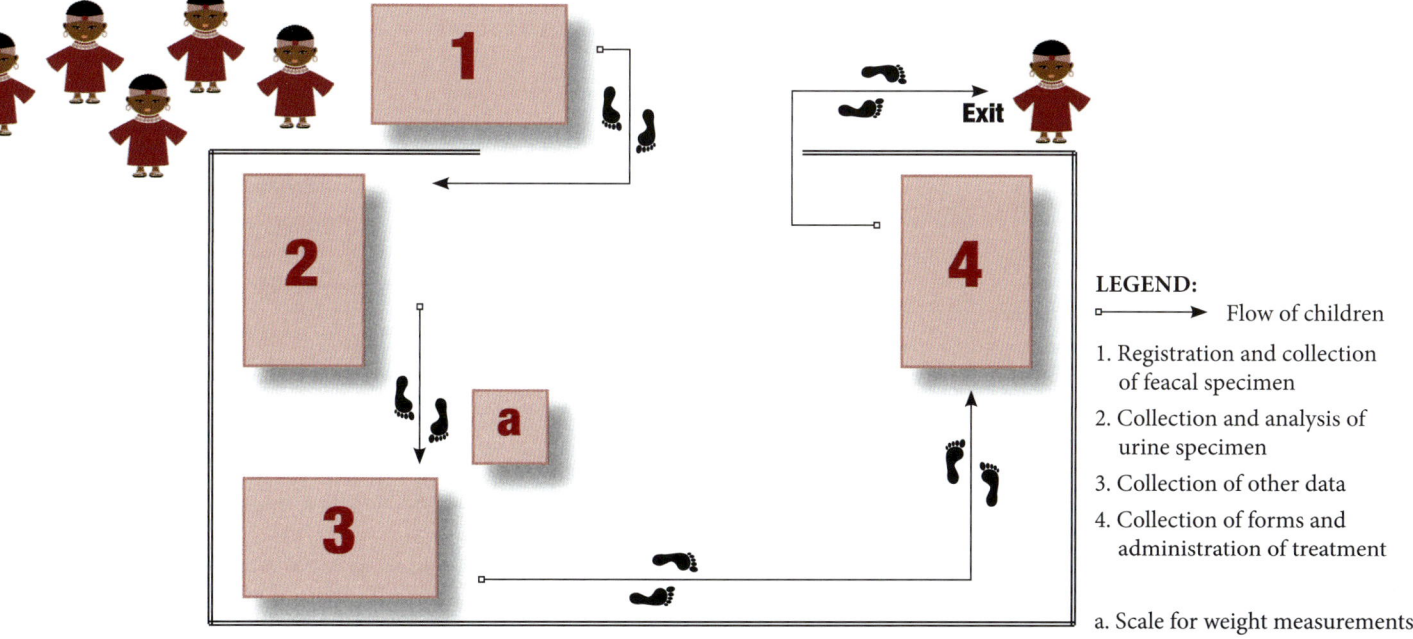

LEGEND:

□——→ Flow of children

1. Registration and collection of feacal specimen
2. Collection and analysis of urine specimen
3. Collection of other data
4. Collection of forms and administration of treatment

a. Scale for weight measurements

5.4.2   Urine examination

There are two options for the diagnosis of *S. haematobium*:

- Detection of eggs in urine. The filtration technique (WHO, 1991) involves the microscopic examination of a filter used to collect the eggs of *S. haematobium* from 10 ml of urine. The urinary excretion of these eggs follows a daily rhythm, with a peak around noon. Urine specimens for filtration are therefore best collected between 10:00 and 14:00 (10 a.m. and 2 p.m.). Physical exercise combined with fluid intake has been shown to significantly increase egg output (Doehring et al., 1983); it is therefore useful to ask the schoolchildren to do some short physical exercise before collecting the urine specimens.

- Detection of haematuria. Visible haematuria may be detected by direct observation of the urine specimen, which appears reddish in colour. This is an important sign of heavy infection with *S. haematobium* (Savioli et al., 1990). Detection of microhaematuria requires the use of a reagent strip that is dipped into the urine specimen for about 1 minute and then compared with a colour scale supplied with the strips. Intensity of infection can be estimated according to the quantity of blood detected by the strip. Since haematuria tends to be more consistent than excretion of eggs, the strips can be used at any time of the day. The method is quick, easy to perform, and highly sensitive and specific (Savioli et al., 1989).

The Kato–Katz, filtration techniques, and reagent strips, are easy to use in field situations:

- Simple equipment is needed: a light microscope, the Kato–Katz kit and the urine filters or strips.
- Most material for the Kato–Katz (templates, slides) and urine filtration (filter holders) may be reused after thorough washing.
- Urine filtration and reagent strips allow diagnosis while the child is still present, allowing any necessary treatment to be given immediately.
- With Kato–Katz kits, slide preparation and examination can be done in the field, immediately after stool collection.

Addresses for procuring this laboratory material and obtaining updated information on costs are given in *Annex 1*.

The appearance and diagnostic features of common intestinal helminths known to infect humans are illustrated in Bench aids for the diagnosis of intestinal parasites (WHO, 1994). The bench aids can be used as a reference by laboratory technicians during training activities and in laboratory diagnosis; an electronic copy of the document is available at the WHO/NTD web site (see *Annex 1*).

Table 5.1 Classes of intensity for soil-transmitted helminths and schistosomes[a]

Parasite	Light-intensity infections[b]	Moderate-intensity infections[b]	Heavy-intensity infections[b]
A. lumbricoides	1–4 999 epg	5 000–49 999 epg	≥50 000 epg
T. trichiura	1–999 epg	1 000–9 999 epg	≥10 000 epg
Hookworms	1–1 999 epg	2 000–3 999 epg	≥4 000 epg
S. mansoni	1–99 epg	100–399 epg	≥400 epg
S. haematobium	1–50 eggs/10 ml of urine		>50 eggs/10 ml of urine (or visible haematuria)

[a] WHO, 2002.
[b] epg = eggs per gram of faeces.

5.4.3 Safety procedures

Team members are advised to wear latex gloves during the collection, preparation and reading of the microscopic slides of stool and urine specimens. Any material contaminated with stool or urine should be cleaned with water and soap and then soaked in sodium hypochlorite solution (or other suitable disinfectant). The containers and slides can then be rinsed and dried for reuse or disposed of by incineration.

5.5 Analysis of data

5.5.1 Individual results

Laboratory examination during the survey will classify each individual as testing positive or negative for each species of helminth egg. Individuals can also be classified according to intensity of infection (no infection; or light, moderate or heavy intensity of infection), measured in terms of eggs per gram (epg) of faeces[1] and, for urinary schistosomiasis, eggs per 10 ml of urine. The classes of intensity proposed for the classification of *individual* infection, based on the report of the WHO Expert Committee (WHO, 2002), are presented in *Table 5.1*.

5.5.2 Community results

The prevalence of infection (the percentage of infected individuals in a population) is calculated as follows:

$$Prevalence = \frac{\text{Number of subjects testing positive}}{\text{Number of subjects investigated}} \times 100$$

The prevalence can be calculated separately for each parasite or as prevalence of any STH (or any schistosome) infection.

The *intensity of infection at community* level (which provides an indication of the morbidity caused by the infection) can be expressed in different ways, including mean arithmetic epg and mean geometric epg, but the most comprehensive and operational way is to present the intensity of infection by the proportions of individuals in each class of intensity (Montresor, 2007).

$$\begin{array}{c} Prevalence\ of \\ any\ heavy \\ STH\ infection[2] \end{array} = \frac{\text{Number of subjects heavily infected with any STH}}{\text{Number of subjects investigated}} \times 100$$

Classification of the results into classes of intensity allows an immediate assessment of the proportion of individuals suffering from the severe consequences of the infection and therefore, of the public health relevance of the infections in the community.

Since the first objective of any control programme is to reduce the proportion of heavily infected individuals, this indicator is extremely important for monitoring the progress of the programme. If at all possible, intensity data should be collected in the sentinel sites (see Example 9 in Burkina Faso for the decline in the proportion of individuals in the class of "heavy intensity of infection" over time).

---

[1] With the Kato–Katz technique, the epg value is obtained by multiplying the number of eggs counted on the slide by a factor that varies according to the size of the template used. WHO recommends the use of a template holding 41.7 mg of faeces, which corresponds to a multiplication factor of 24.

[2] The same formula applies for calculating the prevalence of heavy schistosome infection.

References

Belizario VY Jr et al. (2009). Sentinel surveillance of soil-transmitted helminthiasis in selected local government units in the Philippines. *Asia-Pacific Journal of Public Health*, 21:26–42.

Doehring E, Feldmeier H, Daffalla AA (1983). Day-to-day variation and circadian rhythm of egg excretion in urinary schistosomiasis in the Sudan. *Annals of Tropical Medicine and Parasitology*, 77:587–594.

Koukounari A et al. (2007). *Schistosoma haematobium* infection and morbidity before and after large-scale administration of praziquantel in Burkina Faso. *Journal of Infectious Diseases*, 196:659–669.

Lwanga SK, Lemeshow S (1991). *Sample size determination in health studies*. Geneva, World Health Organization.

Montresor A (2007). Arithmetic or geometric means of eggs per gram are not appropriate indicators to estimate the impact of control measures in helminth infections. *Transactions of the Royal Society of Tropical Medicine and Hygiene*, 101:773–776.

Savioli L et al. (1989). Control of morbidity due to *Schistosoma haematobium* on Pemba Island; selective population chemotherapy of schoolchildren with haematuria to identify high-risk localities. *Transactions of the Royal Society of Tropical Medicine and Hygiene*, 83:805–810.

Savioli L et al. (1990). Control of morbidity due to *Schistosoma haematobium* on Pemba Island: egg excretion and hematuria as indicators of infection. *American Journal of Tropical Medicine and Hygiene*, 43:289–295.

Touré S et al. (2008). Two-year impact of single praziquantel treatment on infection in the national control programme on schistosomiasis in Burkina Faso. *Bulletin of the World Health Organization*, 86:780–787.

WHO (1991). *Basic laboratory methods in medical parasitology*. Geneva, World Health Organization.

WHO (1994). *Bench aids for the diagnosis of intestinal parasites*. Geneva, World Health Organization.

WHO (2002). *Prevention and control of schistosomiasis and soil-transmitted helminthiasis. Report of a WHO Expert Committee*. Geneva, World Health Organization (WHO Technical Report Series, No. 912).

In order to report regularly on progress towards the 2010 target (WHA 54.19), WHO has established a databank to collect annual data on the number of children receiving treatment against schistosomiasis and STH infections

Photograph by WHO

OPPORTUNITIES

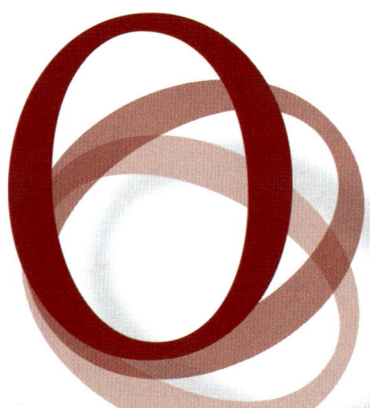

In order to report regularly on progress towards the 2010 target (WHA 54.19), WHO has established a databank to collect annual data on the number of children receiving treatment against schistosomiasis and STH infections (see *Annex 1*).

Progress in coverage from 2005 to 2009 is illustrated in *Figure 6.1*, which indicates that, in 2009, approximately 8% of school-age children in endemic areas received appropriate treatment for schistosomiasis and 30% for STH infections. A growing number of partners are now focusing attention on the prevention and control of neglected tropical diseases, attracted by the simplicity and low cost of the interventions and the considerable health benefits that can be achieved.

Donors include:

- bilateral organizations (Japan International Cooperation Agency, United Kingdom Department for International Development, United States Agency for International Development);
- pharmaceutical companies (Bayer, GlaxoSmithKline, Johnson & Johnson, Merck KGaA);
- philanthropic foundations; (Bill & Melinda Gates Foundation, Children's Investment Fund Foundation, Global Network for Neglected Tropical Diseases, Ivo

de Carneri Foundation, Task Force for Global Health);
- multilateral agencies (UNICEF, World Bank, WFP);
- universities (Centre for Neglected Tropical Diseases at Liverpool School of Tropical Medicine, George Washington University, London School of Hygiene and Tropical Medicine, McGill University, Sabin Institute, Swiss Tropical Institute);
- nongovernmental organizations focusing on child and maternal health (Helen Keller International, RTI international, Save the Children, World Vision) or specifically on school-based activities targeting STH and schistosome infections (Children Without Worms, Deworm the World, Schistosomiasis Control Initiative).

Contact details and web page links for these partners are included in the list of useful addresses in *Annex 1*. The list will be periodically updated on-line.

As a result of this increase in the financial, technical and intellectual resources available for the control of NTD in general and for school-based control programmes in particular, new deworming initiatives are being planned and initiated every month and existing programmes are being extended over longer periods.

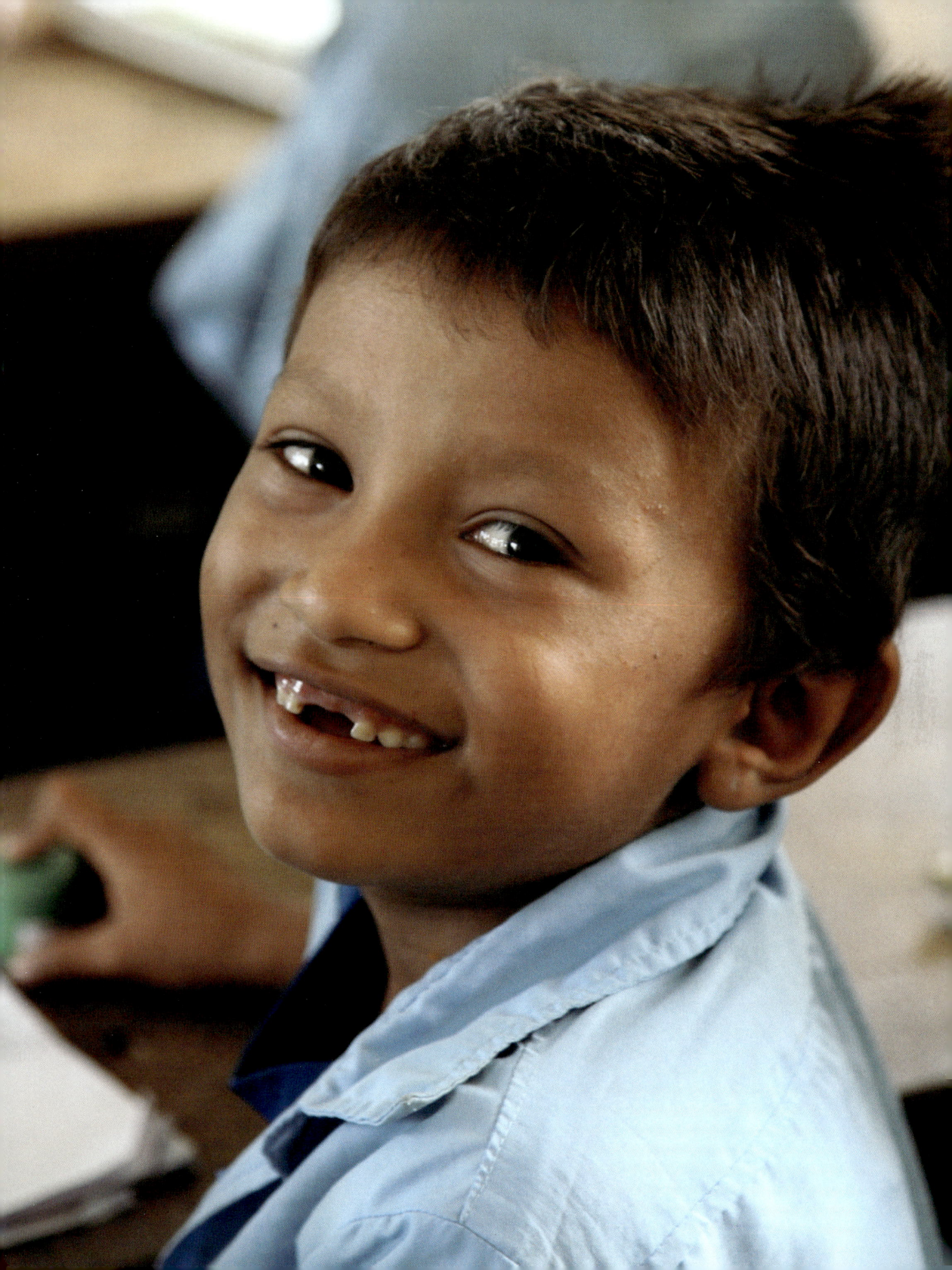

Opportunities

In addition, the experience gained in the application of control measures by national programme managers represents a valuable and growing local resource in terms of the managerial expertise that allows further improvement in efficiency. For the first time in history, it is possible to reduce the disease burden that is attributable to schistosomiasis and STH infections, which has tormented humanity over millennia.

Figure 6.1a Number of people (millions) treated against schistosomiasis, 2005–2009[a]

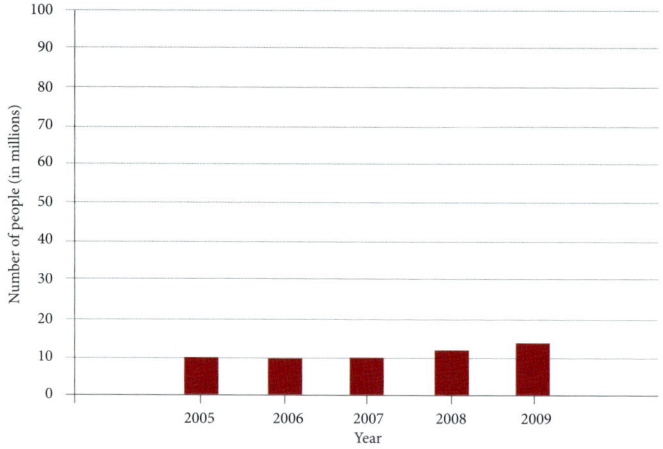

^a Source: WHO (preventive chemotherapy databank).

Figure 6.1b Number of school-age children (millions) treated against soil-transmitted helminth infections, 2003–2009[a]

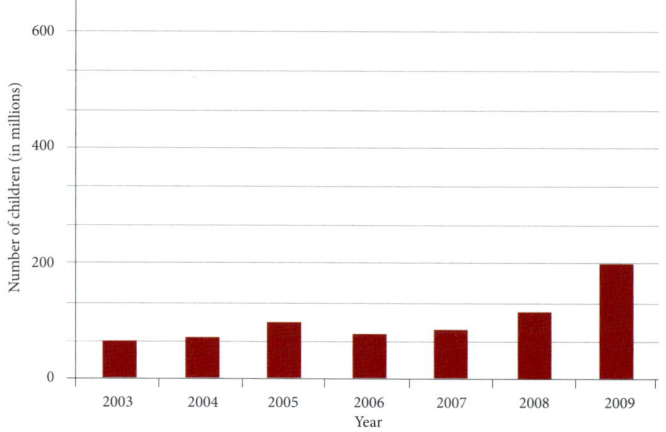

^a Source: WHO (preventive chemotherapy databank).

ANNEXES

Annex 1. List of useful addresses and web links

A1.1 Sources of epidemiological data and information on existing school deworming programmes

WHO/NTD country profiles
WHO has prepared a series of country profiles presenting, for each endemic country, an estimate of the population at risk, epidemiological maps and progress towards reaching the coverage goals. The WHO/NTD country profiles are available at:

http://www.who.int/neglected_diseases/preventive_ chemotherapy/profiles/en/index.html

WHO/NTD databank
In order to report regularly on progress towards the 2010 target, WHO has established a databank of annual data on the number of school-age children and preschool-age children receiving treatment against STH. For each endemic country, the following data are available by year:

- the estimated number of preschool-age and school-age children requiring preventive chemotherapy;
- the number of preschool-age and school-age children reported to have been treated.

The databank is accessible at the WHO/NTD web site:

http://www.who.int/neglected_diseases/preventive_ chemotherapy/sth/en/index.html

Global atlas of helminth infections
The *Global atlas of helminth infections* is an open-access information resource on the distribution of STH and schistosomiasis prepared by the London School of Hygiene and Tropical Medicine, and is available at:

http://www.thiswormyworld.org/

Global atlas on schistosomiasis
The *Global atlas on schistosomiasis* was published in 1987 but remains an extremely useful document today. For each country, a brief overview of the situation, in both French and English, describes:

- the distribution of the infection as derived from epidemiological surveys;
- the climatic and physical conditions in the country, for example, water bodies, that make transmission more likely; and
- any human activities, for example the building of dams or irrigation systems, that increase infection rates.

http://www.who.int/wormcontrol/documents/maps/en/

A1.2 Support for the planning and implementation of deworming programmes in schools

WHO headquarters
Department of Control of Neglected Tropical Diseases (NTD)
Preventive Chemotherapy and Transmission Control (PCT)
World Health Organization
1211 Geneva 27
Switzerland
Tel: +41 22 791 3539 (PCT secretary)
Fax: +41 22 791 4869
E-mail: wormcontrol@who.int
Web site: http://www.who.int/neglected_diseases/en/

Focal points for helminth control in WHO regional offices

- WHO Regional Office for Africa (AFRO)
  Dr Adiele Nkasiobi Onyeze
  E-mail: onyezea@afro.who.int

- WHO Regional Office for the Americas/Pan American Health Organization (AMRO/PAHO)
  Mr Steven K. Ault
  E-mail: aultstev@paho.org

- WHO Regional Office for the Eastern Mediterranean (EMRO)
  Dr Riadh Ben-Ismail
  E-mail: ismailr@emro.who.int

- WHO Regional Office for Europe (EURO)
  Dr Nedret Emiroglu
  E-mail: nem@euro.who.int

- WHO Regional Office for South-East Asia (SEARO)
  Professor A.P. Dash (CDC)
  E-mail: Dasha@searo.who.int

- WHO Regional Office for the Western Pacific (WPRO)
  Dr Eva Maria Christophel
  E-mail: christophele@wpro.who.int

Additional contacts in WHO/HQ

- Nutrition for Health and Development (NHD)
  E-mail: brancaf@who.int

- Prevention of Blindness and Deafness (PBD)
  E-mail: PBD@who.int

A1.3 Additional groups providing support for implementing STH and schistosomiasis control activities

Bilateral organizations

- United Kingdom Department for International Development (DFID)
  http://www.dfid.gov.uk/

- Japan International Cooperation Agency (JICA)
  http://www.jica.go.jp/english/

- United States Agency for International Development (USAID)
  http://www.usaid.gov

Philanthropic foundations

- Bill & Melinda Gates Foundation
  http://www.gatesfoundation.org

- Children's Investment Fund Foundation
  http://www.ciff.org/

- Global Network for Neglected Tropical Diseases
  http://www.globalnetwork.org/

- Ivo de Carneri Foundation
  http://www.fondazionedecarneri.it/

- Task Force for Global Health
  http://www.taskforce.org/

Universities

- Centre for Neglected Tropical Diseases
  Liverpool School of Tropical Medicine
  http://www.lstmliverpool.ac.uk/research/research-environment/centre-for-neglected-tropical-diseases

- Department of Microbiology, Immunology, and Tropical Medicine
  George Washington University
  http://www.gwumc.edu/microbiology/information/index.htm

- London School of Hygiene and Tropical Medicine
  http://www.lshtm.ac.uk/

- McGill University
  http://www.clinepi.mcgill.ca

- Sabin Institute
  http://www.sabin.org/

- Swiss Tropical and Public Health Institute
  http://www.swisstph.ch/

Nongovernmental organizations
- RTI international
  http://www.rti.org

- Save the Children
  http://www.savethechildren.org

- Children Without Worms
  http://www.childrenwithoutworms.org/

- Deworm the World
  http://www.dewormtheworld.org/

- Schistosomiasis Control Initiative (SCI)
  http://www3.imperial.ac.uk/schisto

- WaterAid
  http://www.wateraid.org/

- World Vision
  http://www.wvi.org/

Multilateral organizations
- United Nations Children's Fund (UNICEF)
  http://www.unicef.org

- World Bank, FRESH Initiative
  http://go.worldbank.org/EHK1IVXSV0

- World Bank, Global partnership for education
  http://www.educationfasttrack.org/

- World Food Programme
  http://www.wfp.org/school-meals

A1.4 Information on major drug donation initiatives for benzimidazoles (albendazole or mebendazole) and praziquantel

- GlaxoSmithKline (albendazole)
  http://www.gsk.com/media/pressreleases/2011/2011-pressrelease-616401.htm

- Johnson & Johnson (mebendazole)
  http://www.jnj.com/connect/caring/corporate-giving/preventing-disease/intestinal-worms

- Merck KGaA (praziquantel)
  http://www.merckgroup.com/en/media/extNewsDetail.html?newsId=1FD7AA717642503CC1257964005220E8&newsType=1

- Children Without Worms
  http://www.childrenwithoutworms.org/

- Deworm the World
  http://www.dewormtheworld.org/

A1.5 Companies producing/distributing drugs or laboratory materials

- International Dispensary Association (IDA) – drugs
  http://www.ida.nl/
  E-mail: IDA_sale@euronet.nl

- UNICEF – drugs and laboratory materials
  http://www.unicef.org/supply/index_27571.html

- Vestergaard Frandesen Group – Kato–Katz kits
  http://www.vestergaard-frandsen.com/
  E-mail: sales@vestergaard-frandsen.dk

- Millipore – for filter holders
  http://www.millipore.com/catalogue/module/C160

- Sefar – filters
  http://www.sefar.com
  E-mail: hans-peter.brunner@sefar.ch

- Neolab – hydrophilic cellophane for Kato-Katz
  http://www.neolab.de

A1.6 Assistance with procurement of drugs and other materials

WHO Contractual and Procurement Services (CPS)
Department of Operational Supplies and Services (OSS)
Cluster of General Management (GMG)
World Health Organization
1211 Geneva 27
Switzerland
Fax + 41 22 791 4196 or + 41 22 791 4166
E-mail: procurement@who.int

Current conditions relating to drug procurement through PRS/WHO are the following:

- PRS guarantees best prevailing prices and quality;
- for orders over US$ 70 000, PRS writes out an international tender;
- for orders below US$ 70 000, PRS uses a simplified procedure of competitive bidding;
- PRS charges 3% overhead costs;
- pre-payment is requested and can be made through the WHO country representative;
- payment in local currency can be discussed with the WHO country representative.

A1.7   List of prequalified drug quality control laboratories

An updated list of prequalified laboratories that conduct drug quality control tests is available at:
http://apps.who.int/prequal/lists/PQ_QCLabsList.pdf

A1.8   Examples of health education material

http://www.who.int/intestinal_worms/resources/health_education/en/index.html

A1.9   Links to useful sources (United Nations agencies and partner organizations)

- Assuring safety of preventive chemotherapy interventions for the control of neglected tropical diseases
  http://whqlibdoc.who.int/publications/2011/97892415 02191_eng.pdf

- Bench aids for the diagnosis of intestinal parasites
  http://www.who.int/wormcontrol/documents/benchaids/training_manual/en/

- Basic laboratory methods in medical parasitology
  http://whqlibdoc.who.int/publications/9241544104_(part1).pdf

- Education Management Information System (EMIS)
  http://www.iiep.unesco.org/fileadmin/user_upload/Research_Highlights_Emergencies/Chapter34.pdf

- Haemoglobin concentrations for the diagnosis of anaemia and assessment of severity
  http://www.who.int/vmnis/indicators/haemoglobin.pdf

- International pharmacopoeia
  http://apps.who.int/phint/en/p/about/

- Iron deficiency anaemia: assessment, prevention and control. A guide for programme managers
  http://whqlibdoc.who.int/hq/2001/WHO_NHD_01.3.pdf

- Lymphatic filariasis training documents for the implementation of strategies for the elimination
  http://www.who.int/lymphatic_filariasis/resources/en/

- Operational principles for good pharmaceutical procurement
  http://www.who.int/3by5/en/who-edm-par-99-5.pdf

- Measuring change in nutritional status: guidelines for assessing the nutritional impact of supplementary feeding programmes for vulnerable groups
  http://whqlibdoc.who.int/publications/1983/9241541660.pdf

- Monitoring drug coverage for preventive chemotherapy
  http://whqlibdoc.who.int/publications/2010/9789241599993_eng.pdf

- Preventive chemotherapy in human helminthiasis: coordinated use of anthelminthic drugs in control programmes. A manual for health professionals and programme managers
  http://www.who.int/neglected_diseases/preventive_chemotherapy/pct_manual/en/index.html

- Report of the WHO informal consultation on monitoring of drug efficacy in the control of schistosomiasis and intestinal helminths
  http://whqlibdoc.who.int/hq/1999/WHO_CDS_CPC_SIP_99.1.pdf

- School-based immunization, WHO web page
  http://www.who.int/immunization_delivery/systems_policy/school-based-immunization/en/index.html

- School feeding handbook
  http://www.schoolsandhealth.org/sites/ffe/Key%20Information/WFP%20Basic%20Tools%20-%20School%20Feeding/School%20Feeding%20Handbook.pdf

- Strengthening interventions to reduce helminth infections as an entry point for the development of health promoting schools (WHO Information Series on School Health, Document One)
  http://www.who.int/school_youth_health/media/en/95.pdf

- The sanitation problem: what can and should the health sector do?
  http://www.wateraid.org/documents/the_sanitation_problem__what_can_and_should_the_health_sector_do.pdf

- The schistosomiasis manual
  http://whqlibdoc.who.int/hq/1995/TDR_SER_MSR_95.2.pdf

- Ultrasound in schistosomiasis: a practical guide to the standardized use of ultrasonography for the assessment of schistosomiasis-related morbidity.
  http://apps.who.int/tdr/publications/training-guideline-publications/ultrasound-in-schistosomiasis/pdf/ultrasound-schistosomiasis.pdf

- Water, sanitation and hygiene standards for schools in low-cost settings
  http://www.unicef.org/wash/schools/files/rch_who_standards_2010.pdf

- Weekly Epidemiological Record (WER)
  Every year, WHO publishes in the WER a summary of the number of school-age children and preschool-age children who have received deworming drugs.
  http://www.who.int/wer/en/
  - The WER issue reporting STH deworming data for 2009 is available at:
    http://www.who.int/wer/2011/wer8625.pdf.
  - The WER issue reporting schistosomiasis control data for 2009 is available at:
    http://www.who.int/wer/2011/wer8609/en/index.html

- World Health Assembly resolution 54.19
  http://www.who.int/neglected_diseases/mediacentre/WHA_54.19_Eng.pdf

Annexes

Annex 2. List of materials for parasitological data collection in sentinel sites

The following list of materials is suggested for data collection on 250 children (using a field team of 3 or 4 people):

Materials required	Numbers required	Producer (for addresses see *Annex 1*)
For collecting stool and urine specimens		
Plastic containers[a] (100 ml) with covers for stools	250	
Plastic containers[b] (250 ml) for urine	250	
Permanent-ink marker pens	5	
For analysing specimens		
Microscopes (eyepiece 10x, objectives 10x)	2	International Dispensary Association (IDA)
Microscope slides	250	
Forceps	2	
Disposable gloves (non-sterile)	1 pack of 100	
Kato–Katz kit for 500 stool specimens	1	Vestergaard Frandesen Group
Glycerine	200 ml	
Green malachite powder (optional)	5 g	
Urine reagent strips (blood) or	250	International Dispensary Association
Polycarbonate filters (diameter 13 mm, pore size 12–20 μm)	250	
Polycarbonate filters (pore size 20 μm) and		Sefar Flytis
Filter holders for filtration	50	Swinnex Filter Holder 13 mm Catalogue No. SX00 013 00 Millipore
For cleaning recyclable materials		
Brushes	3	Available locally
Heavy-duty rubber gloves	3 pairs	Available locally
Bucket	2	Available locally
Powdered soap	250 g	Available locally
Sodium hypochlorite (bleach)	3 litres	Available locally
For data registration		
Pencils	10	Available locally
Forms (see Annex 4 and 5)	300	
For treatment		
Mebendazole (500 mg) or Albendazole (400 mg)	To treat not just the classes participating in the survey but the entire school	International Dispensary Association (IDA) UNICEF Supply Division
Praziquantel (600 mg)		
Scales (for praziquantel dosing) (bathroom type for adults)	1	

[a] The stool containers should be plastic to allow for recycling, and should be large enough to allow the child to easily introduce a small quantity (10 g) of stool, using a wooden stick.

[b] If filtration technique is used, the urine container should be large enough to allow the child to collect all the urine, as the eggs of *S. haematobium* tend to be found in the last few drops.

Annex 3. Checklist

Planning the campaign

- ☐ Epidemiological data available that justify the school intervention
- ☐ Agreement reached between partners: Ministry of Education and different managers in the Ministry of Health
- ☐ Initial budget prepared
- ☐ Potential partners consulted (United Nations agencies, nongovernmental organizations, foundations, etc.)
- ☐ Detailed cost estimated
- ☐ Financial gaps identified
- ☐ Financial resources secured
- ☐ Appropriate timing for interventions identified (avoiding school holidays and examination times, religious observance days, periods of intense agricultural work)
- ☐ Programmes conducting similar interventions informed to avoid duplication or waste of resources (e.g. distribution of albendazole to the entire population for the lymphatic filariasis elimination programme)
- ☐ Drugs of good quality ordered in appropriate quantity
- ☐ Customs formalities ascertained and exemptions obtained, if necessary
- ☐ Tablet poles ordered in adequate quantity for distribution of praziquantel
- ☐ Opportunity of joint training discussed among partners
- ☐ Training curriculum agreed upon
- ☐ Mechanism for dispatching drugs and other materials to provinces, districts and schools identified
- ☐ Method of including non-enrolled children identified
- ☐ Mechanisms for collecting forms completed by teachers during drug administration activities identified
- ☐ Communication plan formulated and resourced (including information for families and teachers and emphasis on non-enrolled school-age children)
- ☐ Communication material developed (and pretested)
- ☐ Monitoring tools developed and pretested

Implementing the campaign

- ☐ Training of teachers implemented
- ☐ Teachers informed about reasons for the deworming campaign
- ☐ Teachers consulted about possible timing of the deworming campaign
- ☐ Teachers instructed on how to complete the forms and on the reporting system, including what to do in case of adverse effects
- ☐ Health personnel informed about the campaign and agreement reached about provision of monitoring and support activities
- ☐ Families informed of the reasons for, and timing of, the deworming campaign
- ☐ Drugs dispatched to regions (provinces) with clear instructions regarding onward dispatch to lower levels (districts, schools)
- ☐ Plans for supervisory visits drawn up by central teams

Monitoring the campaign

- ☐ List of indicators identified
- ☐ Periodic collection of parasitological data in sentinel sites planned
- ☐ Discussions held among the different stakeholders about responding to logistic and other possible problems arising during the campaign

Annex 4. School form

SCHISTOSOMIASIS AND SOIL-TRANSMITTED HELMINTHIASES
SCHOOL SURVEY

SCHOOL FORM
to be completed **by the survey team**

School _____   Date [dd/mm/yr]___/___/_____

Region _____   District _____

Total number of forms collected _____   from no. _____ to no _____

I COMPOSITION

Total number of schoolchildren _____   Number of girls in the school _____

Number of classes _____   Number of teachers _____

II WATER

Is there a source of water in the school?   Yes ☐ No ☐

If Yes, type of water source _____

Are there water sources close to the school?   Yes ☐ No ☐

If yes, type of water source _____

III SANITATION

Are there latrines in the school?   Yes ☐ No ☐

Condition of latrines _____

IV HEALTH

Nearest health facility_____

Type _____   Distance _____ km

V TREATMENT

Number of children treated for soil-transmitted helminthiasis:

Enrolled _____   Non-enrolled _____

Number of children treated for schistosomiasis:

Enrolled _____   Non-enrolled _____

SCHISTOSOMIASIS AND SOIL-TRANSMITTED HELMINTHIASES
SCHOOL SURVEY

CHILD FORM
PARASITOLOGICAL/NUTRITIONAL DATA
to be completed **by the survey team**

Date [dd/mm/yr]___/___/_____

I PERSONAL DATA

ID Number_____   School (or village)_____

Name_____   Age_____ (years)   Sexe M □   F □

II NUTRITIONAL DATA

Weight_____ kg   Height_____ cm   Hb_____ g/l

Anaemia   Yes □ No □   Severe anaemia   Yes □ No □

III PARASITOLOGICAL DATA

(a) Stool examination

	eggs/slide	eggs/gram (epg)	Heavy-intensity threshold	Heavy-intensity infection	
				Yes	No
Ascaris lumbricoides			≥50 000 epg		
Trichuris trichiura			≥10 000 epg		
Hookworms			≥4 000 epg		
Schistosoma mansoni/japonicum			≥400 epg		
Other parasites identified:					

(b) Urine, visual examination

	Yes	No
Visible haematuria		
Microhaematuria (reagent strips)		

(c) Urine, examination by microscope

	eggs/10 ml urine	Heavy-intensity threshold	Heavy-intensity infection	
			Yes	No
Schistosoma haematobium (filtration)		>50 eggs/10 ml		

Annex 6. Tally sheet for recording preventive chemotherapy treatments at drug distribution points

Drugs distributed (tick): □ Praziquantel □ Albendazole/Mebendazole □ Ivermectin □ DEC □ Azithromycin

Zone: District: Health unit: Village:

NUMBER OF CHILDREN TREATED

Sex	Male			Female		
Age group	1–4 years	5–14 years	≥15 years	1–4 years	5–14 years	≥15years
	OOOOO OOOOO	OOOOO OOOOO	OOOOO OOOOO	OOOOO OOOOO	OOOOO OOOOO	OOOOO OOOOO
	OOOOO OOOOO	OOOOO OOOOO	OOOOO OOOOO	OOOOO OOOOO	OOOOO OOOOO	OOOOO OOOOO
	OOOOO OOOOO	OOOOO OOOOO	OOOOO OOOOO	OOOOO OOOOO	OOOOO OOOOO	OOOOO OOOOO
	OOOOO OOOOO	OOOOO OOOOO	OOOOO OOOOO	OOOOO OOOOO	OOOOO OOOOO	OOOOO OOOOO
	OOOOO OOOOO	OOOOO OOOOO	OOOOO OOOOO	OOOOO OOOOO	OOOOO OOOOO	OOOOO OOOOO
	OOOOO OOOOO	OOOOO OOOOO	OOOOO OOOOO	OOOOO OOOOO	OOOOO OOOOO	OOOOO OOOOO
	OOOOO OOOOO	OOOOO OOOOO	OOOOO OOOOO	OOOOO OOOOO	OOOOO OOOOO	OOOOO OOOOO
	OOOOO OOOOO	OOOOO OOOOO	OOOOO OOOOO	OOOOO OOOOO	OOOOO OOOOO	OOOOO OOOOO
	OOOOO OOOOO	OOOOO OOOOO	OOOOO OOOOO	OOOOO OOOOO	OOOOO OOOOO	OOOOO OOOOO
	OOOOO OOOOO	OOOOO OOOOO	OOOOO OOOOO	OOOOO OOOOO	OOOOO OOOOO	OOOOO OOOOO
	OOOOO OOOOO	OOOOO OOOOO	OOOOO OOOOO	OOOOO OOOOO	OOOOO OOOOO	OOOOO OOOOO
	OOOOO OOOOO	OOOOO OOOOO	OOOOO OOOOO	OOOOO OOOOO	OOOOO OOOOO	OOOOO OOOOO
Total treated, by age group						
Total treated, by sex						
Total treated (M + F):						

Drugs	Name	Received	Distributed	Lost	Balance

Annex 7. Drug distribution form for enrolled school-age children

SCHISTOSOMIASIS AND SOIL-TRANSMITTED HELMINTHIASES
SCHOOL SURVEY

DRUG DISTRIBUTION FORM FOR <u>ENROLLED</u> SCHOOL-AGE CHILDREN
to be completed by the teacher on each treatment day

School name _____   Location _____   Class _____

Teacher _____   Region _____   District _____

Health education activities performed?   ☐ Yes ☐ No

Describe health education activities on the reverse side of this form.

Names of enrolled children, from class roster	Sex M	Sex F	1st round date __/__/___ PZQ*	1st round date __/__/___ ALB	2nd round date __/__/___ PZQ*	2nd round date __/__/___ ALB	3rd round date __/__/___ PZQ*	3rd round date __/__/___ ALB
1								
2								
3								
4								
5								
6								
7								
8								
9								
10								
11								
12								
13								
14								
15								
16								
17								
18								
19								
20								
21								
22								
23								
24								
25								
Number of children enrolled								
Number of children treated								
Total quantity of drug used								

* For praziquantel (PZQ), indicate the number of tablets given to each child.

Annex 8. Drug distribution form for non-enrolled school-age children

SCHISTOSOMIASIS AND SOIL-TRANSMITTED HELMINTHIASES
SCHOOL SURVEY

DRUG DISTRIBUTION FORM FOR <u>NON-ENROLLED</u> SCHOOL-AGE CHILDREN
to be completed by the teacher on each treatment day

School name _____   Location _____   Date ___ / ___ / _____

Teacher _____   Region _____   District _____

Names of children receiving treatment	Sex		Age	Drug administered	
	M	F		PZQ*	ALB
1					
2					
3					
4					
5					
6					
7					
8					
9					
10					
11					
12					
13					
14					
15					
16					
17					
18					
19					
20					
21					
22					
23					
24					
25					
Number of children treated					
Total quantity of drug used					

* For praziquantel (PZQ), indicate the number of tablets given to each child.

Annex 9. Drug sample collection form

DRUG SAMPLE COLLECTION FORM

Code assigned to sample _____   Date of sample collection [dd/mm/yr] ___/___/_____

Sampling site (facility name, address, contact person) _____

_____

Product name_____

Active ingredient(s) _____

List of excipients _____

_____

Dosage form _____   Strength (e.g. mg/tablet) _____

Primary container (e.g. strips, PVC bottle) _____

Original package size _____

Sample is:

in original sealed package ☐   in original package but not sealed ☐   loose units ☐

Total quantity of sample product at sampling site _____

Quantity collected (specify pack size) _____

Storage conditions at sampling site (give brief description, with temperature and relative humidity data if available)_____

_____

Length of time drug was kept at sampling site _____

Batch number _____   Date of manufacture ___ / ___ /_____   Expiry date ___ / ___ / _____

Name, address and contact details of manufacturer _____

_____

Marketing authorization holder and number _____

Reason for quality testing request _____

_____

Reason original container not provided or opened (if applicable) _____

_____

Any other comments _____

_____

_____

Signature of person collecting the sample _____

Name _____   Date ___ / ___ /_____

Contact details _____

_____

_____

Annexes

Annex 10. Suggested changes in frequency of drug administration after 5–6 years of interventions

After 5-6 years of deworming with good coverage, parasitological indicators collected at sentinel sites normally show a reduced prevalence and intensity of infection in the target population. It is not possible to predict whether this reduction will be permanent or whether infection will return to original levels soon after the interruption of regular treatment.

The table below is intended to help managers of control programmes decide whether and how to reduce the frequency of deworming interventions. Since very few programmes have documented the details of such interventions, the proposed thresholds should be considered only as indications. The following measures apply if the coverage of the intervention has constantly exceeded 75%. If satisfactory coverage has not been reached, the decision to reduce the frequency of interventions should be deferred until coverage is satisfactory.

The thresholds proposed are more restrictive than those given in *Tables 2.2* and *2.3* because prevalence data are collected in situations in which anthelminthic drugs have been administered for several years. In such situations, even a moderate prevalence (of, for example, 20% for STH) indicates that the parasites maintain transmission capacity despite intense drug pressure, and this is predictive of a rapid return to high levels of prevalence if the intervention is interrupted.

Monitoring activities in sentinel sites should continue each year after the frequency of drug administration has been reduced.

If monitoring shows that the prevalence remains low for 4 years despite the reduced frequency of drug administration, a further reduction could be applied. If monitoring indicates that prevalence tends to return to original levels (recrudescence of the infections), reintroduction of the original treatment schedules will be warranted.

In the case of SCH, when prevalence reaches very low levels it is necessary to introduce serological (antigen detection) or molecular (PCR) methods for diagnosis because the classical parasitological methods have low sensitivity in this situation.[1]

These interim suggestions are based on expert opinion and were discussed:

- for STH, during the *Working Group meeting on monitoring and evaluation of preventive chemotherapy* (WHO headquarters, Geneva, Switzerland, 22–23 February 2011);
- for SCH, during the *Informal Consultation on schistosomiasis control* (WHO headquarters, Geneva, Switzerland, 30–31 April 2011).

The suggestions are also valid for deciding the frequency of deworming for STH after the distribution of albendazole has been interrupted, in the context of an LF control programme that normally takes place 5–6 years after the start of interventions (see *section 2.5*).

The table will be updated when new data become available.

[1] Elimination of schistosomiasis from low-transmission areas. Report of a WHO Informal Consultation. Geneva, World Health Organization, 2009 (also available at: http://whqlibdoc.who.int/hq/2009/WHO_HTM_NTD_PCT_2009.2_eng.pdf).

A) Prevalence of SCH

A) Prevalence of SCH	Comment	Suggested frequency of interventions	Additional measures
Over 50%	Prevalence or morbidity is not controlled: intensify frequency of interventions	Intensify the frequency of interventions – check coverage and compliance	Extend coverage to other groups at risk or possibly to the entire population in the area. Reinforce measures for safe water, sanitation and health education
Between 10% and 50%	Prevalence or morbidity has not been sufficiently controlled: maintain frequency of interventions	Maintain treatment of school-age children at previous level for the next 4 years	
Between 1% and 10%	Morbidity is under control but the risk of re-emergence is high: frequency of interventions can be reduced	Administer 1 round of praziquantel every 2 years for the next 4 years	Continue sentinel site monitoring annually (even when the drug is not distributed) to inform managers on possible recrudescence of the infections
Lower than prevalence by standard parasitology	Morbidity is under control with low risk of re-emergence: conduct serological investigation to focalise the intervention: reduce frequency of intervention where serology/PCR is negative and focalise intervention in areas where it is positive	No treatment is needed in areas where serology is negative. Administer 1 round of praziquantel every 2 years in areas where serology is positive	Use a more sensitive method for the evaluation of the prevalence (i.e. serology, PCR)

B) Prevalence of STH

B) Prevalence of STH	Comment	Suggested frequency of interventions	Additional measures
Over 50%	Prevalence or morbidity is not controlled: intensify frequency of interventions	Intensify the frequency of interventions – check coverage and compliance	Extend coverage to other groups at risk or possibly to the entire population in the area Reinforce measures for safe water, sanitation and health education
Between 20% and 50%	Prevalence or morbidity has not been sufficiently controlled: maintain frequency of interventions	Maintain treatment of school-age children at previous level for the next 4 years	
Between 10% and 20%	Morbidity is under control but the risk of re-emergence is high: reduce frequency of interventions	Administer 1 round of anthelminthic treatment every year for the next 4 years	Continue sentinel site monitoring annually (even when the drug is not distributed) to inform managers on possible recrudescence of the infections
Between 1% and 10%	Morbidity is under control and the risk of re-emergence is low: reduce the frequency of interventions	Administer 1 round of anthelminthic treatment every 2 years for the next 4 years	
Lower than 1%	No need of preventive chemotherapy	No preventive chemotherapy	

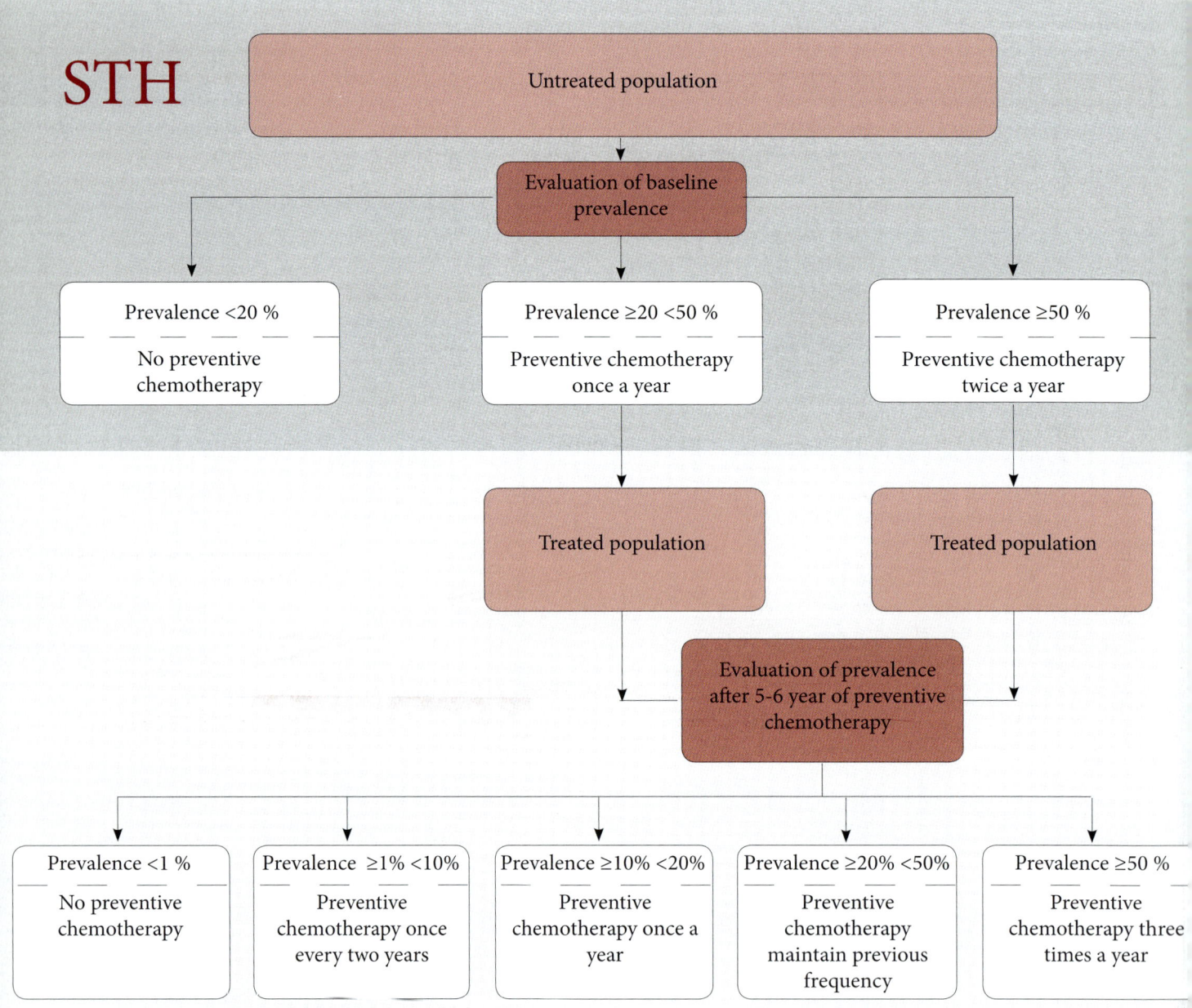

STH

Untreated population

Evaluation of baseline prevalence

Prevalence <20 %	Prevalence ≥20 <50 %	Prevalence ≥50 %
No preventive chemotherapy	Preventive chemotherapy once a year	Preventive chemotherapy twice a year

Treated population

Treated population

Evaluation of prevalence after 5-6 year of preventive chemotherapy

Prevalence <1 %	Prevalence ≥1% <10%	Prevalence ≥10% <20%	Prevalence ≥20% <50%	Prevalence ≥50 %
No preventive chemotherapy	Preventive chemotherapy once every two years	Preventive chemotherapy once a year	Preventive chemotherapy maintain previous frequency	Preventive chemotherapy three times a year

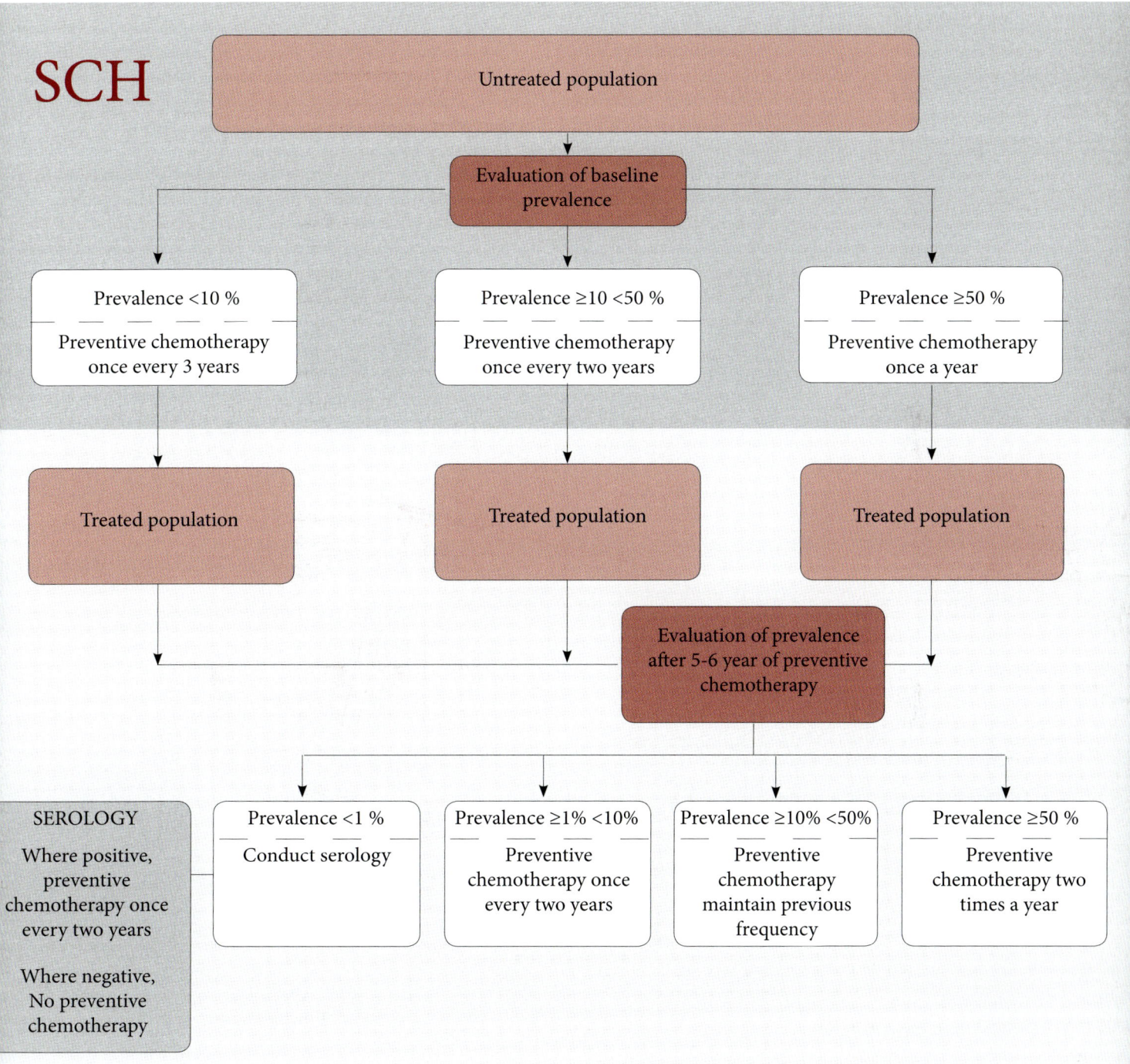

SCH

Untreated population

Evaluation of baseline prevalence

Prevalence <10 %	Prevalence ≥10 <50 %	Prevalence ≥50 %
Preventive chemotherapy once every 3 years	Preventive chemotherapy once every two years	Preventive chemotherapy once a year

Treated population

Treated population

Treated population

Evaluation of prevalence after 5-6 year of preventive chemotherapy

SEROLOGY

Where positive, preventive chemotherapy once every two years

Where negative, No preventive chemotherapy

Prevalence <1 %	Prevalence ≥1% <10%	Prevalence ≥10% <50%	Prevalence ≥50 %
Conduct serology	Preventive chemotherapy once every two years	Preventive chemotherapy maintain previous frequency	Preventive chemotherapy two times a year

Annexes

ANNEXES

Annex 1. List of useful addresses and web links

A1.1 Sources of epidemiological data and information on existing school deworming programmes

WHO/NTD country profiles
WHO has prepared a series of country profiles presenting, for each endemic country, an estimate of the population at risk, epidemiological maps and progress towards reaching the coverage goals. The WHO/NTD country profiles are available at:

http://www.who.int/neglected_diseases/preventive_ chemotherapy/profiles/en/index.html

WHO/NTD databank
In order to report regularly on progress towards the 2010 target, WHO has established a databank of annual data on the number of school-age children and preschool-age children receiving treatment against STH. For each endemic country, the following data are available by year:

– the estimated number of preschool-age and school-age children requiring preventive chemotherapy;
– the number of preschool-age and school-age children reported to have been treated.

The databank is accessible at the WHO/NTD web site:

http://www.who.int/neglected_diseases/preventive_ chemotherapy/sth/en/index.html

Global atlas of helminth infections
The *Global atlas of helminth infections* is an open-access information resource on the distribution of STH and schistosomiasis prepared by the London School of Hygiene and Tropical Medicine, and is available at:

http://www.thiswormyworld.org/

Global atlas on schistosomiasis
The *Global atlas on schistosomiasis* was published in 1987 but remains an extremely useful document today. For each country, a brief overview of the situation, in both French and English, describes:

- the distribution of the infection as derived from epidemiological surveys;
- the climatic and physical conditions in the country, for example, water bodies, that make transmission more likely; and
- any human activities, for example the building of dams or irrigation systems, that increase infection rates.

http://www.who.int/wormcontrol/documents/maps/en/

A1.2   Support for the planning and implementation of deworming programmes in schools

WHO headquarters
Department of Control of Neglected Tropical Diseases (NTD)
Preventive Chemotherapy and Transmission Control (PCT)
World Health Organization
1211 Geneva 27
Switzerland
Tel: +41 22 791 3539 (PCT secretary)
Fax: +41 22 791 4869
E-mail: wormcontrol@who.int
Web site: http://www.who.int/neglected_diseases/en/

Focal points for helminth control in WHO regional offices
- WHO Regional Office for Africa (AFRO)
  Dr Adiele Nkasiobi Onyeze
  E-mail: onyezea@afro.who.int

- WHO Regional Office for the Americas/Pan American Health Organization (AMRO/PAHO)
  Mr Steven K. Ault
  E-mail: aultstev@paho.org

- WHO Regional Office for the Eastern Mediterranean (EMRO)
  Dr Riadh Ben-Ismail
  E-mail: ismailr@emro.who.int

- WHO Regional Office for Europe (EURO)
  Dr Nedret Emiroglu
  E-mail: nem@euro.who.int

- WHO Regional Office for South-East Asia (SEARO)
  Professor A.P. Dash (CDC)
  E-mail: Dasha@searo.who.int

- WHO Regional Office for the Western Pacific (WPRO)
  Dr Eva Maria Christophel
  E-mail: christophele@wpro.who.int

Additional contacts in WHO/HQ
- Nutrition for Health and Development (NHD)
  E-mail: brancaf@who.int

- Prevention of Blindness and Deafness (PBD)
  E-mail: PBD@who.int

A1.3   Additional groups providing support for implementing STH and schistosomiasis control activities

Bilateral organizations
- United Kingdom Department for International Development (DFID)
  http://www.dfid.gov.uk/

- Japan International Cooperation Agency (JICA)
  http://www.jica.go.jp/english/

- United States Agency for International Development (USAID)
  http://www.usaid.gov

Philanthropic foundations
- Bill & Melinda Gates Foundation
  http://www.gatesfoundation.org

- Children's Investment Fund Foundation
  http://www.ciff.org/

- Global Network for Neglected Tropical Diseases
  http://www.globalnetwork.org/

- Ivo de Carneri Foundation
  http://www.fondazionedecarneri.it/

- Task Force for Global Health
  http://www.taskforce.org/

Universities
- Centre for Neglected Tropical Diseases
  Liverpool School of Tropical Medicine
  http://www.lstmliverpool.ac.uk/research/research-environment/centre-for-neglected-tropical-diseases

- Department of Microbiology, Immunology, and Tropical Medicine
  George Washington University
  http://www.gwumc.edu/microbiology/information/index.htm

- London School of Hygiene and Tropical Medicine
  http://www.lshtm.ac.uk/

- The sanitation problem: what can and should the
  health sector do?
  http://www.wateraid.org/documents/the_sanitation_
  problem__what_can_and_should_the_health_sector_
  do.pdf

- The schistosomiasis manual
  http://whqlibdoc.who.int/hq/1995/TDR_SER_MSR_
  95.2.pdf

- Ultrasound in schistosomiasis: a practical guide to the
  standardized use of ultrasonography for the
  assessment of schistosomiasis-related morbidity.
  http://apps.who.int/tdr/publications/training-
  guideline-publications/ultrasound-in-schistosomiasis/
  pdf/ultrasound-schistosomiasis.pdf

- Water, sanitation and hygiene standards for schools in
  low-cost settings
  http://www.unicef.org/wash/schools/files/rch_who_
  standards_2010.pdf

- Weekly Epidemiological Record (WER)
  Every year, WHO publishes in the WER a summary
  of the number of school-age children and preschool-
  age children who have received deworming drugs.
  http://www.who.int/wer/en/
  - The WER issue reporting STH deworming data for
    2009 is available at:
    http://www.who.int/wer/2011/wer8625.pdf.
  - The WER issue reporting schistosomiasis control
    data for 2009 is available at:
    http://www.who.int/wer/2011/wer8609/en/
    index.html

- World Health Assembly resolution 54.19
  http://www.who.int/neglected_diseases/
  mediacentre/WHA_54.19_Eng.pdf

Current conditions relating to drug procurement through PRS/WHO are the following:

- PRS guarantees best prevailing prices and quality;
- for orders over US$ 70 000, PRS writes out an international tender;
- for orders below US$ 70 000, PRS uses a simplified procedure of competitive bidding;
- PRS charges 3% overhead costs;
- pre-payment is requested and can be made through the WHO country representative;
- payment in local currency can be discussed with the WHO country representative.

A1.7 List of prequalified drug quality control laboratories

An updated list of prequalified laboratories that conduct drug quality control tests is available at:
http://apps.who.int/prequal/lists/PQ_QCLabsList.pdf

A1.8 Examples of health education material

http://www.who.int/intestinal_worms/resources/health_education/en/index.html

A1.9 Links to useful sources (United Nations agencies and partner organizations)

- Assuring safety of preventive chemotherapy interventions for the control of neglected tropical diseases
  http://whqlibdoc.who.int/publications/2011/9789241502191_eng.pdf

- Bench aids for the diagnosis of intestinal parasites
  http://www.who.int/wormcontrol/documents/benchaids/training_manual/en/

- Basic laboratory methods in medical parasitology
  http://whqlibdoc.who.int/publications/9241544104_(part1).pdf

- Education Management Information System (EMIS)
  http://www.iiep.unesco.org/fileadmin/user_upload/Research_Highlights_Emergencies/Chapter34.pdf

- Haemoglobin concentrations for the diagnosis of anaemia and assessment of severity
  http://www.who.int/vmnis/indicators/haemoglobin.pdf

- International pharmacopoeia
  http://apps.who.int/phint/en/p/about/

- Iron deficiency anaemia: assessment, prevention and control. A guide for programme managers
  http://whqlibdoc.who.int/hq/2001/WHO_NHD_01.3.pdf

- Lymphatic filariasis training documents for the implementation of strategies for the elimination
  http://www.who.int/lymphatic_filariasis/resources/en/

- Operational principles for good pharmaceutical procurement
  http://www.who.int/3by5/en/who-edm-par-99-5.pdf

- Measuring change in nutritional status: guidelines for assessing the nutritional impact of supplementary feeding programmes for vulnerable groups
  http://whqlibdoc.who.int/publications/1983/9241541660.pdf

- Monitoring drug coverage for preventive chemotherapy
  http://whqlibdoc.who.int/publications/2010/9789241599993_eng.pdf

- Preventive chemotherapy in human helminthiasis: coordinated use of anthelminthic drugs in control programmes. A manual for health professionals and programme managers
  http://www.who.int/neglected_diseases/preventive_chemotherapy/pct_manual/en/index.html

- Report of the WHO informal consultation on monitoring of drug efficacy in the control of schistosomiasis and intestinal helminths
  http://whqlibdoc.who.int/hq/1999/WHO_CDS_CPC_SIP_99.1.pdf

- School-based immunization, WHO web page
  http://www.who.int/immunization_delivery/systems_policy/school-based-immunization/en/index.html

- School feeding handbook
  http://www.schoolsandhealth.org/sites/ffe/Key%20Information/WFP%20Basic%20Tools%20-%20School%20Feeding/School%20Feeding%20Handbook.pdf

- Strengthening interventions to reduce helminth infections as an entry point for the development of health promoting schools (WHO Information Series on School Health, Document One)
  http://www.who.int/school_youth_health/media/en/95.pdf

- McGill University
  http://www.clinepi.mcgill.ca

- Sabin Institute
  http://www.sabin.org/

- Swiss Tropical and Public Health Institute
  http://www.swisstph.ch/

Nongovernmental organizations
- RTI international
  http://www.rti.org

- Save the Children
  http://www.savethechildren.org

- Children Without Worms
  http://www.childrenwithoutworms.org/

- Deworm the World
  http://www.dewormtheworld.org/

- Schistosomiasis Control Initiative (SCI)
  http://www3.imperial.ac.uk/schisto

- WaterAid
  http://www.wateraid.org/

- World Vision
  http://www.wvi.org/

Multilateral organizations
- United Nations Children's Fund (UNICEF)
  http://www.unicef.org

- World Bank, FRESH Initiative
  http://go.worldbank.org/EHK1IVXSV0

- World Bank, Global partnership for education
  http://www.educationfasttrack.org/

- World Food Programme
  http://www.wfp.org/school-meals

A1.4 Information on major drug donation initiatives for benzimidazoles (albendazole or mebendazole) and praziquantel

- GlaxoSmithKline (albendazole)
  http://www.gsk.com/media/pressreleases/2011/2011-pressrelease-616401.htm

- Johnson & Johnson (mebendazole)
  http://www.jnj.com/connect/caring/corporate-giving/preventing-disease/intestinal-worms

- Merck KGaA (praziquantel)
  http://www.merckgroup.com/en/media/extNewsDetail.html?newsId=1FD7AA717642503CC1257964005220E8&newsType=1

- Children Without Worms
  http://www.childrenwithoutworms.org/

- Deworm the World
  http://www.dewormtheworld.org/

A1.5 Companies producing/distributing drugs or laboratory materials

- International Dispensary Association (IDA) – drugs
  http://www.ida.nl/
  E-mail: IDA_sale@euronet.nl

- UNICEF – drugs and laboratory materials
  http://www.unicef.org/supply/index_27571.html

- Vestergaard Frandesen Group – Kato–Katz kits
  http://www.vestergaard-frandsen.com/
  E-mail: sales@vestergaard-frandsen.dk

- Millipore – for filter holders
  http://www.millipore.com/catalogue/module/C160

- Sefar – filters
  http://www.sefar.com
  E-mail: hans-peter.brunner@sefar.ch

- Neolab – hydrophilic cellophane for Kato-Katz
  http://www.neolab.de

A1.6 Assistance with procurement of drugs and other materials

WHO Contractual and Procurement Services (CPS)
Department of Operational Supplies and Services (OSS)
Cluster of General Management (GMG)
World Health Organization
1211 Geneva 27
Switzerland
Fax + 41 22 791 4196 or + 41 22 791 4166
E-mail: procurement@who.int

Annex 2. List of materials for parasitological data collection in sentinel sites

The following list of materials is suggested for data collection on 250 children (using a field team of 3 or 4 people):

Materials required	Numbers required	Producer (for addresses see *Annex 1*)
For collecting stool and urine specimens		
Plastic containers[a] (100 ml) with covers for stools	250	
Plastic containers[b] (250 ml) for urine	250	
Permanent-ink marker pens	5	
For analysing specimens		
Microscopes (eyepiece 10x, objectives 10x)	2	International Dispensary Association (IDA)
Microscope slides	250	
Forceps	2	
Disposable gloves (non-sterile)	1 pack of 100	
Kato–Katz kit for 500 stool specimens	1	Vestergaard Frandesen Group
Glycerine	200 ml	
Green malachite powder (optional)	5 g	
Urine reagent strips (blood) or	250	International Dispensary Association
Polycarbonate filters (diameter 13 mm, pore size 12–20 µm)	250	
Polycarbonate filters (pore size 20 µm) and		Sefar Flytis
Filter holders for filtration	50	Swinnex Filter Holder 13 mm Catalogue No. SX00 013 00 Millipore
For cleaning recyclable materials		
Brushes	3	Available locally
Heavy-duty rubber gloves	3 pairs	Available locally
Bucket	2	Available locally
Powdered soap	250 g	Available locally
Sodium hypochlorite (bleach)	3 litres	Available locally
For data registration		
Pencils	10	Available locally
Forms (see Annex 4 and 5)	300	
For treatment		
Mebendazole (500 mg) or Albendazole (400 mg)	To treat not just the classes participating in the survey but the entire school	International Dispensary Association (IDA) UNICEF Supply Division
Praziquantel (600 mg)		
Scales (for praziquantel dosing) (bathroom type for adults)	1	

[a] The stool containers should be plastic to allow for recycling, and should be large enough to allow the child to easily introduce a small quantity (10 g) of stool, using a wooden stick.

[b] If filtration technique is used, the urine container should be large enough to allow the child to collect all the urine, as the eggs of *S. haematobium* tend to be found in the last few drops.

Annex 3. Checklist

Planning the campaign

- ☐ Epidemiological data available that justify the school intervention
- ☐ Agreement reached between partners: Ministry of Education and different managers in the Ministry of Health
- ☐ Initial budget prepared
- ☐ Potential partners consulted (United Nations agencies, nongovernmental organizations, foundations, etc.)
- ☐ Detailed cost estimated
- ☐ Financial gaps identified
- ☐ Financial resources secured
- ☐ Appropriate timing for interventions identified (avoiding school holidays and examination times, religious observance days, periods of intense agricultural work)
- ☐ Programmes conducting similar interventions informed to avoid duplication or waste of resources (e.g. distribution of albendazole to the entire population for the lymphatic filariasis elimination programme)
- ☐ Drugs of good quality ordered in appropriate quantity
- ☐ Customs formalities ascertained and exemptions obtained, if necessary
- ☐ Tablet poles ordered in adequate quantity for distribution of praziquantel
- ☐ Opportunity of joint training discussed among partners
- ☐ Training curriculum agreed upon
- ☐ Mechanism for dispatching drugs and other materials to provinces, districts and schools identified
- ☐ Method of including non-enrolled children identified
- ☐ Mechanisms for collecting forms completed by teachers during drug administration activities identified
- ☐ Communication plan formulated and resourced (including information for families and teachers and emphasis on non-enrolled school-age children)
- ☐ Communication material developed (and pretested)
- ☐ Monitoring tools developed and pretested

Implementing the campaign

- ☐ Training of teachers implemented
- ☐ Teachers informed about reasons for the deworming campaign
- ☐ Teachers consulted about possible timing of the deworming campaign
- ☐ Teachers instructed on how to complete the forms and on the reporting system, including what to do in case of adverse effects
- ☐ Health personnel informed about the campaign and agreement reached about provision of monitoring and support activities
- ☐ Families informed of the reasons for, and timing of, the deworming campaign
- ☐ Drugs dispatched to regions (provinces) with clear instructions regarding onward dispatch to lower levels (districts, schools)
- ☐ Plans for supervisory visits drawn up by central teams

Monitoring the campaign

- ☐ List of indicators identified
- ☐ Periodic collection of parasitological data in sentinel sites planned
- ☐ Discussions held among the different stakeholders about responding to logistic and other possible problems arising during the campaign

SCHISTOSOMIASIS AND SOIL-TRANSMITTED HELMINTHIASES
SCHOOL SURVEY

SCHOOL FORM
to be completed **by the survey team**

School _____   Date [dd/mm/yr]___/___/_____

Region _____   District _____

Total number of forms collected _____   from no. _____ to no _____

I COMPOSITION

Total number of schoolchildren _____   Number of girls in the school _____

Number of classes _____   Number of teachers _____

II WATER

Is there a source of water in the school?   Yes ☐ No ☐

If Yes, type of water source _____

Are there water sources close to the school?   Yes ☐ No ☐

If yes, type of water source _____

III SANITATION

Are there latrines in the school?   Yes ☐ No ☐

Condition of latrines _____

IV HEALTH

Nearest health facility_____

Type _____   Distance _____ km

V TREATMENT

Number of children treated for soil-transmitted helminthiasis:

Enrolled _____   Non-enrolled _____

Number of children treated for schistosomiasis:

Enrolled _____   Non-enrolled _____

SCHISTOSOMIASIS AND SOIL-TRANSMITTED HELMINTHIASES
SCHOOL SURVEY

CHILD FORM
PARASITOLOGICAL/NUTRITIONAL DATA
to be completed **by the survey team**

Date [dd/mm/yr]____/____/_____

I PERSONAL DATA

ID Number_____   School (or village)_____

Name_____   Age_____ (years)   Sexe M □   F □

II NUTRITIONAL DATA

Weight_____ kg   Height_____ cm   Hb_____ g/l

Anaemia   Yes □ No □   Severe anaemia   Yes □ No □

III PARASITOLOGICAL DATA

(a) Stool examination

	eggs/slide	eggs/gram (epg)	Heavy-intensity threshold	Heavy-intensity infection	
				Yes	No
Ascaris lumbricoides			≥50 000 epg		
Trichuris trichiura			≥10 000 epg		
Hookworms			≥4 000 epg		
Schistosoma mansoni/japonicum			≥400 epg		
Other parasites identified:					

(b) Urine, visual examination

	Yes	No
Visible haematuria		
Microhaematuria (reagent strips)		

(c) Urine, examination by microscope

	eggs/10 ml urine	Heavy-intensity threshold	Heavy-intensity infection	
			Yes	No
Schistosoma haematobium (filtration)		>50 eggs/10 ml		

Annex 6. Tally sheet for recording preventive chemotherapy treatments at drug distribution points

Drugs distributed (tick): ☐ Praziquantel ☐ Albendazole/Mebendazole ☐ Ivermectin ☐ DEC ☐ Azithromycin

Zone: District: Health unit: Village:

NUMBER OF CHILDREN TREATED

Sex	Male				Female			
Age group	1–4 years	5–14 years	≥15 years	1–4 years	≥15 years	5–14 years	≥15years	
	00000 00000	00000 00000	00000 00000	00000 00000	00000 00000	00000 00000	00000 00000	
	00000 00000	00000 00000	00000 00000	00000 00000	00000 00000	00000 00000	00000 00000	
	00000 00000	00000 00000	00000 00000	00000 00000	00000 00000	00000 00000	00000 00000	
	00000 00000	00000 00000	00000 00000	00000 00000	00000 00000	00000 00000	00000 00000	
	00000 00000	00000 00000	00000 00000	00000 00000	00000 00000	00000 00000	00000 00000	
	00000 00000	00000 00000	00000 00000	00000 00000	00000 00000	00000 00000	00000 00000	
	00000 00000	00000 00000	00000 00000	00000 00000	00000 00000	00000 00000	00000 00000	
	00000 00000	00000 00000	00000 00000	00000 00000	00000 00000	00000 00000	00000 00000	
	00000 00000	00000 00000	00000 00000	00000 00000	00000 00000	00000 00000	00000 00000	
	00000 00000	00000 00000	00000 00000	00000 00000	00000 00000	00000 00000	00000 00000	
	00000 00000	00000 00000	00000 00000	00000 00000	00000 00000	00000 00000	00000 00000	
	00000 00000	00000 00000	00000 00000	00000 00000	00000 00000	00000 00000	00000 00000	
	00000 00000	00000 00000	00000 00000	00000 00000	00000 00000	00000 00000	00000 00000	
	00000 00000	00000 00000	00000 00000	00000 00000	00000 00000	00000 00000	00000 00000	
Total treated, by age group								
Total treated, by sex								
Total treated (M + F):								

Drugs	Name	Received	Distributed	Lost	Balance

Annex 7. Drug distribution form for enrolled school-age children

SCHISTOSOMIASIS AND SOIL-TRANSMITTED HELMINTHIASES
SCHOOL SURVEY

DRUG DISTRIBUTION FORM FOR <u>ENROLLED</u> SCHOOL-AGE CHILDREN
to be completed by the teacher on each treatment day

School name _____   Location _____   Class _____
Teacher _____   Region _____   District _____

Health education activities performed?   ☐ Yes ☐ No
Describe health education activities on the reverse side of this form.

| Names of enrolled children, from class roster | Sex | | Drug administered | | | | | |
| | M | F | 1st round date __/__/___ | | 2nd round date __/__/___ | | 3rd round date __/__/___ | |
			PZQ*	ALB	PZQ*	ALB	PZQ*	ALB
1								
2								
3								
4								
5								
6								
7								
8								
9								
10								
11								
12								
13								
14								
15								
16								
17								
18								
19								
20								
21								
22								
23								
24								
25								
Number of children enrolled								
Number of children treated								
Total quantity of drug used								

* For praziquantel (PZQ), indicate the number of tablets given to each child.

Annex 8. Drug distribution form for non-enrolled school-age children

SCHISTOSOMIASIS AND SOIL-TRANSMITTED HELMINTHIASES
SCHOOL SURVEY

DRUG DISTRIBUTION FORM FOR <u>NON-ENROLLED</u> SCHOOL-AGE CHILDREN
to be completed by the teacher on each treatment day

School name _____   Location _____   Date ___ / ___ / _____
Teacher _____   Region _____   District _____

Names of children receiving treatment	Sex		Age	Drug administered	
	M	F		PZQ*	ALB
1					
2					
3					
4					
5					
6					
7					
8					
9					
10					
11					
12					
13					
14					
15					
16					
17					
18					
19					
20					
21					
22					
23					
24					
25					
Number of children treated					
Total quantity of drug used					

* For praziquantel (PZQ), indicate the number of tablets given to each child.

Annex 9. Drug sample collection form

DRUG SAMPLE COLLECTION FORM

Code assigned to sample _____   Date of sample collection [dd/mm/yr] ___/___/_____

Sampling site (facility name, address, contact person) _____
_____

Product name_____

Active ingredient(s) _____

List of excipients _____
_____

Dosage form _____   Strength (e.g. mg/tablet) _____

Primary container (e.g. strips, PVC bottle) _____

Original package size _____

Sample is:
in original sealed package ☐   in original package but not sealed ☐   loose units ☐

Total quantity of sample product at sampling site _____

Quantity collected (specify pack size) _____

Storage conditions at sampling site (give brief description, with temperature and relative humidity data if available)_____
_____

Length of time drug was kept at sampling site _____

Batch number _____   Date of manufacture ___ / ___ /_____   Expiry date ___ / ___ / _____

Name, address and contact details of manufacturer _____
_____

Marketing authorization holder and number _____

Reason for quality testing request _____
_____

Reason original container not provided or opened (if applicable) _____
_____

Any other comments _____
_____
_____

Signature of person collecting the sample _____

Name _____   Date ___ / ___ / _____

Contact details _____
_____
_____

Annex 10. Suggested changes in frequency of drug administration after 5–6 years of interventions

After 5-6 years of deworming with good coverage, parasitological indicators collected at sentinel sites normally show a reduced prevalence and intensity of infection in the target population. It is not possible to predict whether this reduction will be permanent or whether infection will return to original levels soon after the interruption of regular treatment.

The table below is intended to help managers of control programmes decide whether and how to reduce the frequency of deworming interventions. Since very few programmes have documented the details of such interventions, the proposed thresholds should be considered only as indications. The following measures apply if the coverage of the intervention has constantly exceeded 75%. If satisfactory coverage has not been reached, the decision to reduce the frequency of interventions should be deferred until coverage is satisfactory.

The thresholds proposed are more restrictive than those given in *Tables 2.2* and *2.3* because prevalence data are collected in situations in which anthelminthic drugs have been administered for several years. In such situations, even a moderate prevalence (of, for example, 20% for STH) indicates that the parasites maintain transmission capacity despite intense drug pressure, and this is predictive of a rapid return to high levels of prevalence if the intervention is interrupted.

Monitoring activities in sentinel sites should continue each year after the frequency of drug administration has been reduced.

If monitoring shows that the prevalence remains low for 4 years despite the reduced frequency of drug administration, a further reduction could be applied. If monitoring indicates that prevalence tends to return to original levels (recrudescence of the infections), reintroduction of the original treatment schedules will be warranted.

In the case of SCH, when prevalence reaches very low levels it is necessary to introduce serological (antigen detection) or molecular (PCR) methods for diagnosis because the classical parasitological methods have low sensitivity in this situation.[1]

These interim suggestions are based on expert opinion and were discussed:

- for STH, during the *Working Group meeting on monitoring and evaluation of preventive chemotherapy* (WHO headquarters, Geneva, Switzerland, 22–23 February 2011);
- for SCH, during the *Informal Consultation on schistosomiasis control* (WHO headquarters, Geneva, Switzerland, 30–31 April 2011).

The suggestions are also valid for deciding the frequency of deworming for STH after the distribution of albendazole has been interrupted, in the context of an LF control programme that normally takes place 5–6 years after the start of interventions (see *section 2.5*).

The table will be updated when new data become available.

---

[1] Elimination of schistosomiasis from low-transmission areas. Report of a WHO Informal Consultation. Geneva, World Health Organization, 2009 (also available at: http://whqlibdoc.who.int/hq/2009/WHO_HTM_NTD_PCT_2009.2_eng.pdf).

Decision trees

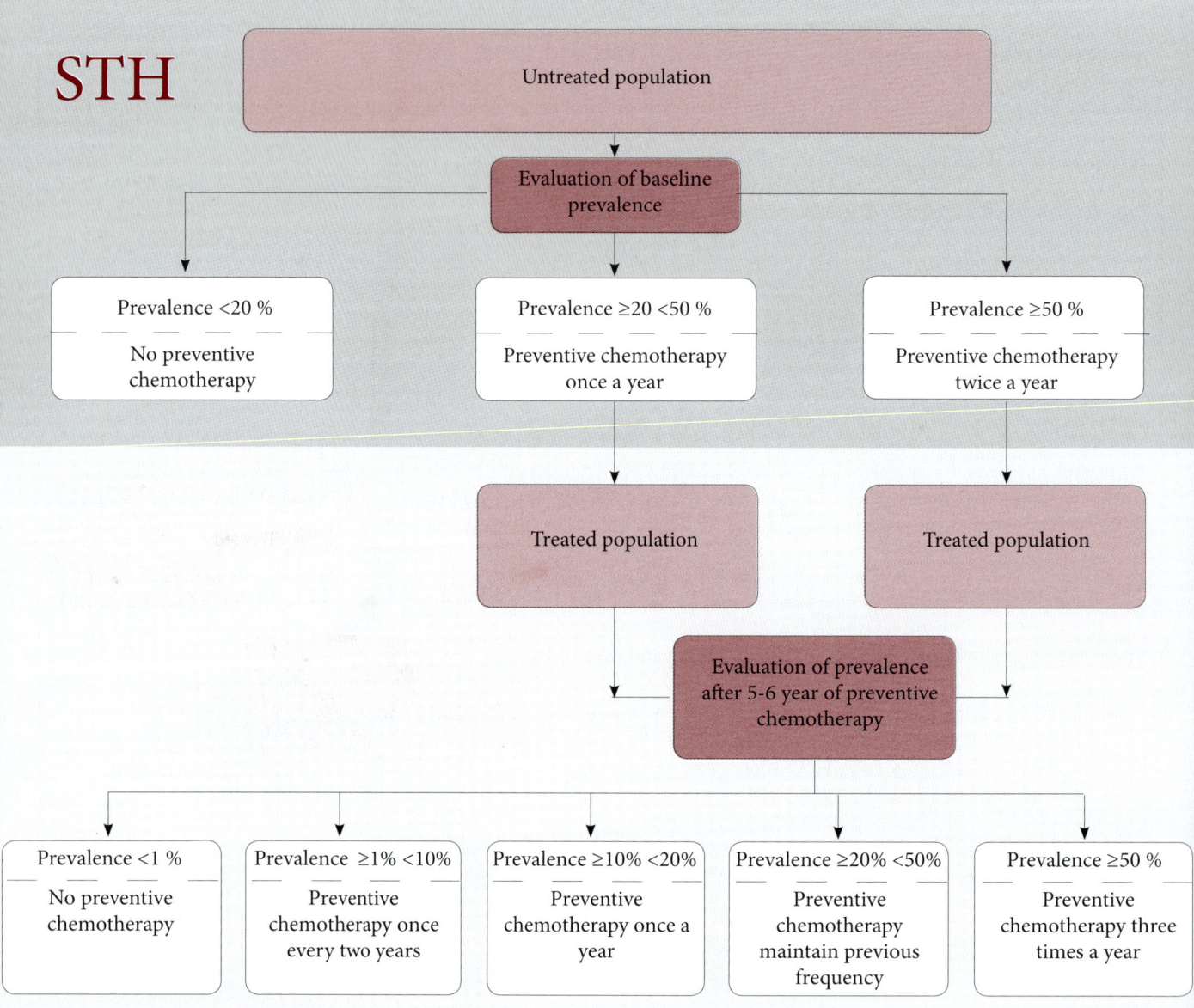

STH

Untreated population

Evaluation of baseline prevalence

Prevalence <20 %

No preventive chemotherapy

Prevalence ≥20 <50 %

Preventive chemotherapy once a year

Prevalence ≥50 %

Preventive chemotherapy twice a year

Treated population

Treated population

Evaluation of prevalence after 5-6 year of preventive chemotherapy

Prevalence <1 %

No preventive chemotherapy

Prevalence ≥1% <10%

Preventive chemotherapy once every two years

Prevalence ≥10% <20%

Preventive chemotherapy once a year

Prevalence ≥20% <50%

Preventive chemotherapy maintain previous frequency

Prevalence ≥50 %

Preventive chemotherapy three times a year

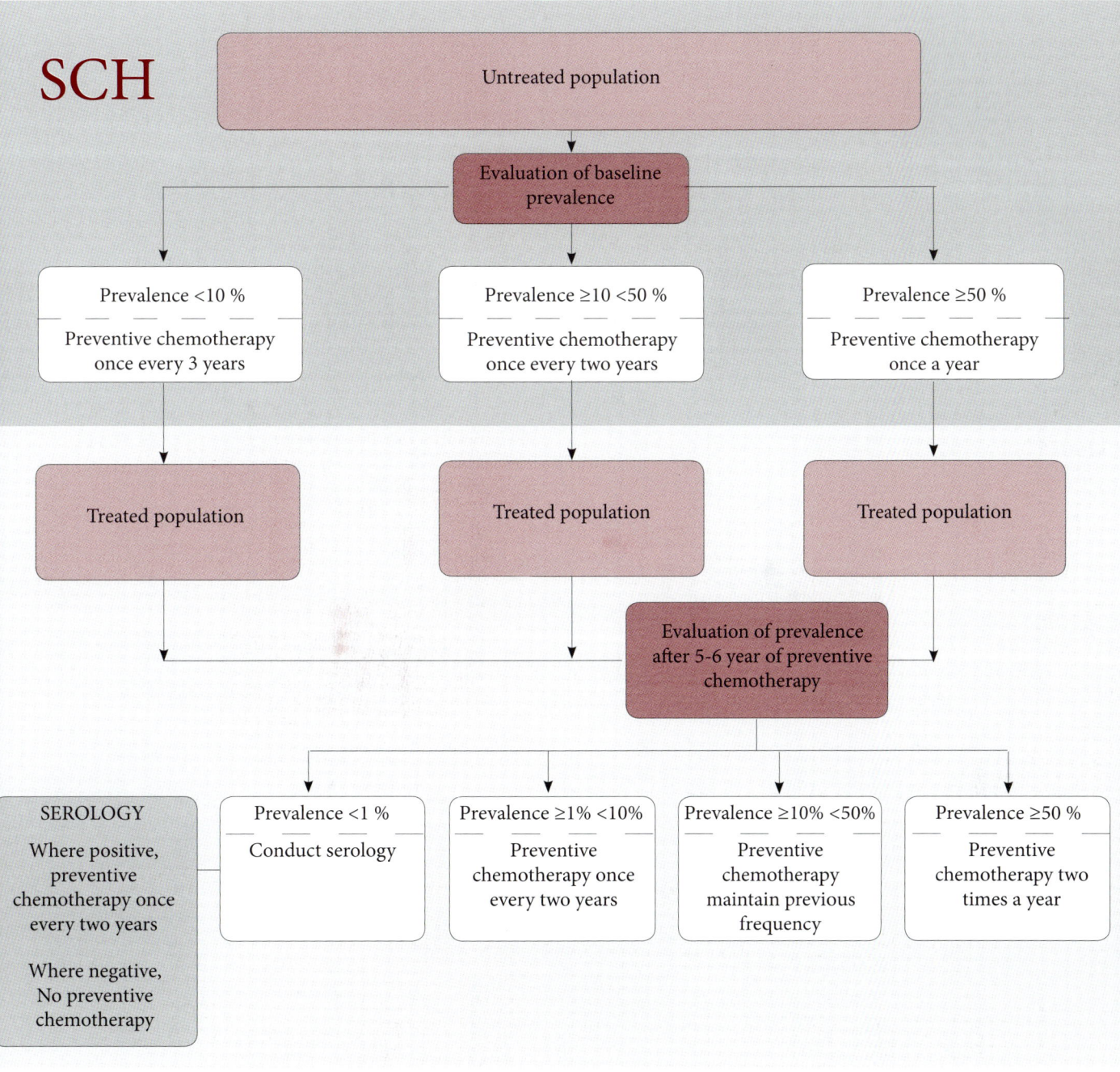

SCH

Untreated population

↓

Evaluation of baseline prevalence

Prevalence <10 %	Prevalence ≥10 <50 %	Prevalence ≥50 %
Preventive chemotherapy once every 3 years	Preventive chemotherapy once every two years	Preventive chemotherapy once a year

Treated population   Treated population   Treated population

Evaluation of prevalence after 5-6 year of preventive chemotherapy

SEROLOGY

Where positive, preventive chemotherapy once every two years

Where negative, No preventive chemotherapy

Prevalence <1 %	Prevalence ≥1% <10%	Prevalence ≥10% <50%	Prevalence ≥50 %
Conduct serology	Preventive chemotherapy once every two years	Preventive chemotherapy maintain previous frequency	Preventive chemotherapy two times a year

A) Prevalence of SCH

Prevalence of SCH	Comment	Suggested frequency of interventions	Additional measures
Over 50%	Prevalence or morbidity is not controlled: intensify frequency of interventions	Intensify the frequency of interventions – check coverage and compliance	Extend coverage to other groups at risk or possibly to the entire population in the area. Reinforce measures for safe water, sanitation and health education
Between 10% and 50%	Prevalence or morbidity has not been sufficiently controlled: maintain frequency of interventions	Maintain treatment of school-age children at previous level for the next 4 years	
Between 1% and 10%	Morbidity is under control but the risk of re-emergence is high: frequency of interventions can be reduced	Administer 1 round of praziquantel every 2 years for the next 4 years	Continue sentinel site monitoring annually (even when the drug is not distributed) to inform managers on possible recrudescence of the infections
Lower than prevalence by standard parasitology	Morbidity is under control with low risk of re-emergence: conduct serological investigation to focalise the intervention: reduce frequency of intervention where serology/PCR is negative and focalise intervention in areas where it is positive	No treatment is needed in areas where serology is negative. Administer 1 round of praziquantel every 2 years in areas where serology is positive	Use a more sensitive method for the evaluation of the prevalence (i.e. serology, PCR)

B) Prevalence of STH

Prevalence of STH	Comment	Suggested frequency of interventions	Additional measures
Over 50%	Prevalence or morbidity is not controlled: intensify frequency of interventions	Intensify the frequency of interventions – check coverage and compliance	Extend coverage to other groups at risk or possibly to the entire population in the area Reinforce measures for safe water, sanitation and health education
Between 20% and 50%	Prevalence or morbidity has not been sufficiently controlled: maintain frequency of interventions	Maintain treatment of school-age children at previous level for the next 4 years	
Between 10% and 20%	Morbidity is under control but the risk of re-emergence is high: reduce frequency of interventions	Administer 1 round of anthelminthic treatment every year for the next 4 years	Continue sentinel site monitoring annually (even when the drug is not distributed) to inform managers on possible recrudescence of the infections
Between 1% and 10%	Morbidity is under control and the risk of re-emergence is low: reduce the frequency of interventions	Administer 1 round of anthelminthic treatment every 2 years for the next 4 years	
Lower than 1%	No need of preventive chemotherapy	No preventive chemotherapy	